BET
RELATIO

You may also be interested in the following Vermilion titles:

After the Affair by Julia Cole
Loving in Later Life by Marj Thoburn and Suzy Powling
Sex in Loving Relationships by Sarah Litvinoff
Starting Again by Sarah Litvinoff
Staying Together by Susan Quilliam
Step-Families by Suzie Hayman
Stop Arguing Start Talking by Susan Quilliam

To obtain a copy, simply telephone TBS Direct on 01206 255800

BETTER RELATIONSHIPS

Practical ways to make your love last

SARAH LITVINOFF

relate

VERMILION
LONDON

For my daughter Jemilah, my nephews Julian and Lucian and my brother Aaron:
in the hope that this book will help you build the loving and
lasting relationships that you all deserve.

1 3 5 7 9 10 8 6 4 2

Copyright © 1991 Sarah Litvinoff and Relate
Sarah Litvinoff and Relate have asserted their moral right to be identified
as the authors of this work in accordance with the Copyright, Designs
and Patents Act 1988.

All rights reserved. No part of this publication may be reproduced, stored
in a retrieval system, or transmitted in any form or by any means, electronic,
mechanical, photocopying or otherwise without the prior permission of the
copyright owners.

First published in 1992 by Vermilion
This edition published in 2001 by Vermilion,
an imprint of Ebury Press, Random House,
20 Vauxhall Bridge Road, London SW1V 2SA
www.randomhouse.co.uk

Random House Australia (Pty) Limited
20 Alfred Street, Milsons Point, Sydney,
New South Wales 2061, Australia

Random House New Zealand Limited
18 Poland Road, Glenfield,
Auckland 10, New Zealand

Random House South Africa (Pty) Limited
Endulini, 5a Jubilee Road, Parktown 2193, South Africa

The Random House Group Limited Reg. No. 954009

Papers used by Vermilion are natural, recyclable products made from wood
grown in sustainable forests.

Printed and bound in Great Britain by
Cox & Wyman Ltd, Reading, Berks

A CIP catalogue record for this book is available from the British Library.

ISBN 0 09 185670 1

CONTENTS

TASKS, QUIZZES AND TALKING POINTS

Throughout the text there are boxes consisting of tasks, quizzes and talking points. A few of these are actual tasks used by Relate counsellors; the others have been especially designed by the author to help you discover things about yourself and each other that would usually emerge during counselling.

Many of the tasks require pen and paper. You will be making lists or notes under various headings. The quizzes can be answered on the page, although you might like to make a copy of some of them so that you and your partner can complete them separately. The talking points raise issues that it would be interesting or useful for you to discuss together, or pick up on a point in the text that you might want to think about further.

It is hoped that you will complete many of these together as a couple, but you should only do so if you are both keen. You can also gain useful insights by doing them alone.

ACKNOWLEDGEMENTS

With grateful thanks to the chairperson of Relate, Ann Leck, a counsellor herself, who read the manuscript as it was being written and made helpful comments. Also to Pauline Batchelor, formerly publications manager of Relate, who helped so much in determining the form the book should take.

Thanks are also due to the following counsellors who provided the backbone of the book by sharing their experiences of clients, and to the employees of Relate who were involved in the book at various stages: Laurel Aarons, Angela Allen, Hilary Andrews, Lyn Bailey, Anita Blum, Val Brewin, Eleanor Briggs, Ann Bryan, Christine Buerk, Pamela Cavendish, Heather Clark, Jan Clark, Alison Clegg, Simon Coles, Jay Davies, Aileen Dempsey, Martin Dodd, Jaci Elliott, Vicky Erich, Helen Evans, Kathy Fox, Judy Goldby, Linda Griffiths, Alan Gudgin, Lizzy Harrison-Cripps, Carolyn Meller, Anne Healey, Gillian Hill, Sue Kennedy, Trish Lebus, Liz Lynch, Peter McCabe, Sue Mervyn Jones, David Mills, Jan Needham, Liz Newnham, Melanie Pany, Sylvia Payne, Shirley Pinfold, Mary Read, Gillina Richardson, Linda Shore, Zelda West-Meads. Olive Whittington, Carol Wine.

Thank you to Henneke Sharif for compiling the organisations list in the Further Help Section.

FOREWORD

Problems can sometimes threaten to overwhelm a relationship. Help from a skilled counsellor allows people to sort out their own feelings and untangle the problems, and to learn skills which will help them cope with future difficulties in a constructive way. This is the rewarding work which the charity Relate is dedicated to – helping people develop their relationships creatively.

Each stage of life brings its own challenge. The life changes attendant on marriage itself – having children, moving house, changing jobs, retirement, all of these – are normal. Some changes are unexpected. Relate helps people to cope with these transitions as they are happening and to equip them with the skills they need to deal with life changes in the future.

Much of Relate's energy is directed towards helping people think about the cornerstones upon which relationships are built and how these can be fostered and maintained over time. Building a strong relationship needs the ability to communicate and to negotiate and manage conflict as well as sexual and physical intimacy. The ability of each partner to put the other first, a willingness to see things from the other's point of view, even when not agreeing with them and an enjoyment of each other's company – these qualities cement a relationship.

It is never too late to learn. It is never too late to brighten up a relationship. *The Relate Guide to Better Relationships* will help you to do just that. The wisdom, sensitivity and skill of the Relate counsellors is encompassed in this highly readable and practical guide. With 60 years' cumulative experience of couple counselling, the experts at Relate know how to overcome difficulties and create a strong, long-lasting relationship. *The Relate Guide to Better Relationships,* complete with quizzes, tasks, discussion points and case histories, explains how to make your love last.

The response to the first edition was wonderful, with over 50,000 copies sold. This new edition includes a fully revised chapter on sex, explaining how it changes over the years, its problems, its joys, and how to make it better.

The Relate Guide to Better Relationships has already made Relate's vast and unique body of experience accessible to thousands of people. We are delighted to welcome this new edition and through it extend our support to many more couples as they build better relationships.

Marj Thoburn
Head of Services to Couples
Relate National

You can find the telephone number of your local Relate centre by looking in the telephone directory under 'Relate' or 'Marriage Guidance'. The national office is at Herbert Gray College, Little Church Street, Rugby CV21 3AP; Tel. 01788 573241

1

ALL YOU NEED IS LOVE

With love comes heartache. This is a fact of life and not as negative as it seems at first. If you don't care deeply for someone disagreements and problems will only be a passing annoyance. The more someone matters to you, the more you will mind when things between you go wrong.

The problems that arise in every partnership test your love – but they can also add to it. The heartache love brings can eventually increase your love. Relate counsellors know that happiness in a relationship does not depend on harmony. Meeting problems together and in the right way deepens love, and couples who learn to tackle differences positively can survive even serious crises. But they can do more than just survive. Working through problems together so that there is no winner or loser has a transforming effect on love. It gives it strength and flexibility and allows you to trust in its power to unite you. Love that has never been tested is more fragile. Problems can be a good thing.

If that is true, why do so many couples break up? Some do at almost the first sign of trouble; others, to the astonishment and grief of family and friends, part after many years – even decades – of marriage. Others cling together forever when clearly there is no love: when struggles and problems have not deepened their love but have curdled it, turning it to bitterness and dislike. These cases show how unresolved problems are disruptive and damaging.

But most things worth having are gained through a great deal of effort and concentration. A deep, lasting, enriching love must be the most precious thing we can have in our lives. It starts, usually, with a wonderful explosion of emotion, passion and excitement. Whether it will burn itself out like a magnificent firework or develop into the kind of strong and fundamental love that we all need depends on how we approach the bad times.

Problems can be good. But only if you both know how to deal with them. That means bringing the best of yourself to the issue: your wisdom and sense of humour, your generosity and respect for each other, your tolerance and your commitment to the relationship. It means patience and courage, sometimes over a long period. This is a tall order, perhaps the most difficult thing you will ever do – but do it right and it will be by far the most rewarding. If it were easy Relate would not exist and no one would need to read this book.

Some people can't or won't ever put this kind of effort into love and therefore will miss out on the richest and most satisfying experience it is possible to have. This book is for those of you who are prepared to do all you can to make your love work but don't know how. It contains practical advice from the counsellors on ways to tackle difficulties and real case-histories from the counsellors' notes.

Much of counselling work involves showing couples how to tackle their problems. Every problem, large or small, challenges you with two possible outcomes: you can diminish your love or strengthen it. There is no magic involved in taking the right course, but many couples who have learnt from counselling feel that the effect in their lives has been magical. Counselling, and this book, can present you with much of the raw material you need to make your relationship the best it can be. But you then have to do the work. This work is never wasted. Learning to handle love and the problems that result from it will make you a stronger and more confident person, as well as benefiting your relationship.

Most of this book looks at the problems that can arise in a relationship. But what about those heady days when problems don't seem to matter – when you are madly in love? What makes you fall in love with someone? Is there anything you should know about yourself or your loved one right at the beginning that will make things easier for you later on? These questions and others are tackled in this chapter and the two that follow.

A 'PERFECT RELATIONSHIP'

At heart most people are looking for their perfect relationship, not one that is just all right or better than most. Once you are in a relationship you will probably be prepared for some compromise, to endure difficulties and disappointments, but a part of you might continue to believe that it shouldn't be necessary, that in a perfect relationship true love should be effortless. If this strikes a chord in you, ask yourself what it is that you imagine a perfect relationship to be. For many people it is an almost mystical union – physical, mental, spiritual and emotional, in which your partner supplies everything you could wish for, harmoniously, for ever.

The reason this image persists is that most of us have a taste of it when we fall in love. The feelings generated by falling in love are some of the most intense we will ever feel. They have been compared to the euphoria of drugs or drink, and like these chemical highs 'in love' feelings drown out other thoughts and sensations. Part of your mind may know that all is not quite right, but the imperfections don't seem to matter. But, as with drugs or drink, these feelings wear off eventually. Yet the tantalising memory of this golden period remains

Real relationships have to leave this fantasy behind. The pity is that some people can't see that in fact the best relationships provide something far more valuable than this romantic fog. When you are 'in love' you are completely wrapped up with the other person in an intoxicatingly exclusive and exciting one-ness. This union would be suffocating and limiting if it continued – but it can't last. Any change in you or your circumstances (even a happy one, such as getting married) has the effect of breaking the spell – slowly, perhaps, but inevitably.

In the best relationships love is a strong invisible bond, flexible and elastic like muscle fibre, which allows each of you to develop as individuals. Some difficult events can stretch it very thin but, again like muscle, using it strengthens it.

Partner is a word often used by journalists who don't want to specify whether they are talking about a marriage partner or a lover or whether a man or a woman is involved. But it is a very good word in its own right. A good relationship is a creative developing *partnership*. A good relationship has ups and downs, and uses them to change and develop. The best relationships can meet almost any challenge and use the experience positively.

A crisis can highlight the value of the relationship, showing you how much it means to you. It can prove how good you are at coping or it can force you to find new ways to cope. All Relate counsellors have stories to tell about couples who have dealt with problems seemingly so intractable that it is difficult to see how the relationship could have survived. Couples in strong relationships find new commitment during these times and go on to feel that they have gained from the experience.

One such example is Alison and Mike. They came for counselling after a profoundly tragic experience: their second child had been born with a heart defect and had died in hospital a few months after birth. It was during this time that Mike told Alison that he had been having an affair with her best friend. The affair was over but Alison was bitterly hurt and didn't know how to cope with the anger she felt for Mike while she was grieving for her lost child, or whether she would ever be able trust him again.

Counselling revealed some of the patterns that had led to this crisis. Mike's background had left him with feelings of failure and a need to be looked after almost like a child. He had been jealous of their first child who had received more 'mothering' from Alison than he had. The death of his second child made him feel guilty – he had an irrational feeling that somehow he should have been able to prevent it – and he felt bad that he had resented Alison's grief for having taken her away from him. Alison herself had problems trusting men because her own father had had many affairs. She did 'mother' Mike, but in a controlling way. Her sadness made her vulnerable and suddenly she needed Mike to look after *her*. Neither of them were good at expressing their feelings.

Knowing that Mike's affair was simply a search for some alleviation of his grief and a need for someone to concentrate lovingly on him during this ordeal provided an opening for counselling, as did the insight that Alison's understandably strong negative feelings and her domination of Mike were a barrier to them moving forward.

But knowing the reasons wasn't enough, however. What the counsellor found was that both partners had a strong commitment to each other and a willingness to change their behaviour if it would make the relationship better. By the end of the counselling she was able to see that their union was stronger than it had ever been – that what they had learned would make their relationship better as the years went on. Alison and Mike agreed. There were still great feelings of sadness about their lost child, but in every other way there was improvement. They felt they had learned important lessons for the future, and they knew that as a result of understanding themselves and one another better they loved each other more deeply than before.

So what had happened? In this case the counsellor had used tasks to help them get to know themselves and to change their ways of behaving. We will go into these in more detail in the chapter on Communication, but will look at them briefly here as they applied to Alison and Mike.

The first task consisted of spending an hour together twice a week, talking about themselves. For the first half hour Alison would talk about herself and her feelings while Mike listened without interrupting. Then they would switch over and Mike would talk about himself. On the second day Mike would be the one to start.

The rules were strict: they could only talk about themselves – not about the other person or the relationship. They had to talk about their emotions, their needs, and how they coped with their feelings – or didn't cope with them. At the end of the session they were not to discuss what had been said until they saw the counsellor.

The first surprise for Alison was how difficult it was for her to listen to Mike without interrupting. Mike was surprised that he was able to find enough things to say to fill half an hour. It was a joy for him not to be interrupted and to know that Alison was not allowed to comment.

This exercise helped them so much that they wanted to continue it for several weeks. Mike began to see that he had a right to feel whatever he did, and Alison learned to avoid trying to influence what he thought or felt. She began to understand what his affair really meant and why he had found it difficult to look after her during her grief. For his part, instead of switching off, Mike became more able to cope with Alison's sadness and feelings of vulnerability because he understood them better.

The next task was to help them meet each other's needs and to increase intimacy. They had got into a pattern of nagging or rowing about what the other did or wanted to do. For instance, Mike would announce that he was going to the pub with a friend: Alison would then complain that he never spent time with her or their son. On alternate days, therefore, they had to ask one another for something they wanted the other to do for them (within limits that they both agreed beforehand – they couldn't ask for anything they knew the other would hate).

The first time they tried this Mike, who had been digging the garden, asked Alison to massage his aching shoulders. Alison's immediate reponse was, 'Oh I don't think the counsellor meant that sort of thing – she meant something a lot deeper than that, intimacy is about more important things.' Mike was upset and didn't ask for anything else – so neither did Alison when it came to her turn. When they next saw the counsellor they reported that the exercise had failed. After they had talked it through, however, Alison was able to see that she was in the habit of thinking that Mike's needs were unimportant.

At the next counselling session they were able to report that it had been a successful week. They had been able to ask one another for whatever they wanted and both had responded gladly. For the first time they were thinking about what they needed and why, telling each other clearly and respecting each other's wishes.

They found they wanted quite simple things. Alison might say, 'I would like us to decide now what we can do together as a family on Saturday so that it doesn't just come and go.' If they had different ideas about how to spend Saturday they would agree to take it in turns to carry them out. They were listening to each other much more carefully and were able to share the responsibility for making the relationship happy.

By the time they had finished the counselling they were handling their relationship in such different ways that they felt confident they would be able to meet any other problems that came up. These simple tasks meant they had become much more in tune with each other and found daily life together happy and pleasant. Most of all they were both developing as people: Mike was growing up now that he knew he couldn't expect Alison to look after him or tell him what to do, and Alison felt able to look to Mike for support when she needed it rather than always being in charge. As the counsellor says, 'The changes they made seem simple but can be quite difficult. They worked really hard because they wanted their relationship to last and they both changed. Many couples aren't ready to put in that much effort.'

Understanding that ups and downs are necessary is an important element in making an enduring relationship. One idea that stands in the way of this realisation is the current view of romantic love: what it is, what it means, and how long it should reasonably last. Messages about this from films, pop songs, books and magazines have an effect on all of us, and sometimes stop us seeing the real value in our love relationships.

THE MYTH OF ROMANTIC LOVE

Romantic love is wonderful. Of course it is not simply a myth; it is also a real experience: dizzy, passionate, exciting and intoxicating. To be romantically in love is about the most thrilling thing that can happen to us. The myth is that this heightened romantic state is 'true' love, the best kind of love and – more damaging still – that it can or should last.

It has been said that the search for romantic love and the perfect relationship has filled the space where religion used to be in the lives of millions of people who no longer have much religious faith. Instead of setting their sights on paradise in the next world many people believe they can find it in this one: in the arms of someone who will make them feel forever passionate and ecstatic.

That this is unattainable doesn't stop people believing it, or hoping that it could be true. By no means everyone clings to this belief, but it is part of our culture and it can make ordinary worthwhile love relationships seem humdrum or disappointing.

For those who do have this belief, part of the myth is that this special love will reveal itself in an extraordinary way – and the phenomenom of love at first sight seems to bear this out.

Love at first sight

It does happen. The questions are, why? What sort of love is it? What does it say about you? Does it last? Some of these issues will be looked at in later chapters because they continue to be relevant within individual relationships and to the problems that can arise in them.

But love at first sight as part of the myth of romantic love is important in itself. If you are inclined to believe that it is impossible to know anything about someone at first sight, it follows that if you do fall instantly in love it is a sign that fate has intervened and that you have found 'the one'. But the thunderbolt that can strike 'across a crowded room' is not a purely magical process, it can be analysed.

At the speed of light, too fast for you to be aware of it consciously, you have gathered a lot of information about the person you have seen:

age, physical attractiveness, manner of dressing, posture, way of talking – these are all important clues. The experience you have gained of other people and of life helps you to process these into something you believe to be a true picture of the other person.

Instant falling in love has to do with some part of you being able to recognise your 'type' when you meet it. And what determines your type is affected by factors of which you are hardly aware.

Your type is a composite picture that starts building up from the moment you are born. Bits and pieces of different people go to make up the whole. It includes your parents, your friends, your own face in the mirror, your first crush, people you have admired, people who have stirred up some kind of strong emotion in you. Sometimes your 'type' is destructive and damaging to you and falling in love with such a person can lead to an unhealthy relationship. None of us can properly analyse what goes to make up our types because the process is not conscious. Many factors are deeply buried, a long-forgotten mix of real people, fantasy and experience. But when the person with the right combination appears, your subconscious – and your body – reacts, sometimes instantly, usually without you understanding what has happened.

This dramatic recognition can happen at any time, and by its very nature can be enormously powerful. Instant sexual attraction plays a part in many such encounters, because it is an essential element in a love relationship. But although lust can masquerade as love, the experienced person does know the difference; it is more subtle than that. Sometimes the sexual element is secondary or at least less obvious than other factors, which may in some cases have powerful spiritual, mental or aesthetic qualities.

If you are a great believer in the myth of romantic, fated love you will be more prone to fall in love at first sight. The more romantic you are and the more you believe in instant love the more likely you are to be on the look-out for it.

But is it 'true' love? Because there is a strong element of real subconscious detective work going on whenever you meet anyone, your judgements and feelings are not illusory. In the first ten minutes of talking to someone, his or her clothes, accent, gestures, and manner of speaking will give you a mass of real and relevant information. There is, nevertheless, a strong element of fantasy involved in love at first sight. It tells you much more about yourself, your past experiences and your needs. In believing you know enough to cause you to fall in love you are, to a degree 'inventing' the other person – and ordinary and mundane human characteristics do not enter into the picture. True love is based on real knowledge of the other person's essential self. The main danger lies in believing that only love that happens at first sight is valid.

A couple who demonstrate the almost supernatural power of love at first sight are Elaine and John. They describe their first encounter as a 'recognition', though neither felt strong sexual attraction. They met at a conference in Birmingham – Elaine lived in London and John in Nottingham. John, in his late forties, was married with three children. His marriage was not happy but his sense of commitment and his strong religious faith meant that he had never thought of leaving his wife or having an affair. Yet, he said, the moment he set eyes on Elaine he was aware of thinking, 'That's her!' Elaine, who had just turned forty, was divorced and happily involved with Angus, whom she loved and with whom she had a very good sexual relationship. She said that the moment she saw John she knew that the love she felt for Angus was a small and passing thing. 'All I could see was John, everybody else seemed to fade away. I just felt, "This is it!"'

They did not start an affair – John's beliefs would not allow it – but there followed a compulsive year in which they wrote, spoke on the phone and met whenever they could. Elaine's relationship with Angus finished, and John felt that he must tell his wife about his feelings for Elaine. As a result his marriage – never good – worsened. Their long-distance, non-sexual love affair revealed that they had a strong intellectual affinity, interrupted by explosive disagreements. Despite this, they continued to feel obsessively drawn to each other. Finally John left his wife for Elaine. They believed that as their feelings had continued to remain strong during the year it was evident that they were meant to be together.

Six months into the relationship they were in trouble. As they came to know each other better they found they were complete opposites, with different values, interests and objectives, and radically opposing views on how men and women should live together and divide the chores. They discovered many things about each other that they actively disliked. For a while even this dislike fed the fantasy. Part of the attraction needed the animosity.

As time went on and the intense 'in love' feelings faded, these bad feelings and opposing ideas meant that they were in no position to construct a warmer, more tender kind of love. Each competed to change the other. A period of counselling left them convinced that they could not bridge the gap between them and John returned to his wife.

To begin with Elaine was bitter and distressed. It took a period of counselling on her own before she was able to realise that beneath her initially strong feelings of love for John she had always known that he was wrong for her, but the attraction had allowed her to ignore it. Looking back at her past relationships she saw that all of them had been with men she disliked and could not live with: very similar to her parents, between whom no love was lost. The only exception had been Angus.

With him she had been happy, content, secure and compatible. This state of harmony, being so unusual for her, had made her edgy. With John, 'Mr Wrong', she found a situation that felt so right she couldn't see that it was doomed.

Sometimes the love you experience at first sight endures, sometimes it doesn't. But to endure, it must develop into a different kind of love. It is no less likely to succeed than a relationship begun on another basis – perhaps more likely, as the strong initial mutual attraction means you want to make it work. Whether the love lasts or not partly depends on how closely the essential person resembles that first image you formed. It also depends on whether you have a tendency, like Elaine, to fall in love with the wrong sort of person. But above all, it depends on whether you can recognise that the intense 'in love' feelings will eventually wear off, however right you are for each other.

THE LOVE HANGOVER

The exhilarating feelings of being 'in love' are only temporary, even when they last for months or years. And, again, as with drugs and drink, there is something to pay when the effects wear off.

In romantic love the 'hangover' or 'withdrawal' symptom is disillusionment. It can be compared to looking at a garden scene through binoculars. First you look through them the wrong way, and what you see is the exquisite beautifully coloured whole, too tiny to make out individual detail. Turn the binoculars around and you see these details magnified: the roses are losing their petals, the grass needs mowing, wherever you focus you seem to see signs of neglect or decay. Both these pictures are distortions. Without the binoculars the garden looks lovely, yet it is not perfect and it needs attention.

This is similar to what happens when feeling 'in love' wears off. All those imperfections you couldn't or wouldn't see can no longer be ignored, and because your previous picture was so rosy the shock is greater. As someone once put it: it's not that you now see your loved one warts and all – now you see *only* the warts. Hangovers and drug-withdrawal leave you feeling awful, love-withdrawal can leave you feeling temporarily that your loved one is awful, even when that is far from the truth.

Of course, you eventually recover from the after effects of an 'in-love' phase that has passed, as you do from a hangover. Then you are able to see the other person more realistically, as a normal human being who possesses good and bad qualities and with whom you might want to spend your life.

But some people don't wish to go through the hangover phase to reach the point of recovery. When the image of perfection is disrupted they want to give up. Sometimes this is the right decision: they can see that the former loved one is not right for them and it would never work. There are, however, occasions when it could have worked had the relationship been given the chance.

More often that not you will continue through the hangover phase into a normal, realistic relationship and start to construct a more fundamental kind of love. This is an important phase in building the foundations of a relationship. Only those who feel that this is a second-best sort of love won't enjoy the phase. If you believe 'in love' should last forever you won't be able to value what you have.

LOVE ADDICTION

The belief that being 'in love' *can* last still persists. Stories that centre on love relationships usually cut off before the phase has passed – even Romeo and Juliet's great love-at-first sight encounter would have settled into an everyday relationship given more time.

But the myth is also encouraged by women's magazines and their features on how to recapture the 'magic' or 'excitement' in your relationship – specifically sexually. We will be dealing with that in more detail in the section on sex, but there are some general points to be made.

For most people 'excitement' and 'magic' mean the feelings they experienced during the heady initial stages. Suggesting that these can be recaptured is a con. It can make you feel that you are missing something in your relationship that would be possible to reignite if only you followed the advice.

A relationship can always be improved. You can make it better, more interesting and – yes – more exciting. What you can never do in a mature relationship is recreate the particular kind of excitement you felt when you were first in love. Sex can become better than ever in quality, but it won't have the special tang, the novelty, of first lust. You can never feel as excited about a person you know really well as you can about a new, mysterious lover with whom you are besotted and about whom there is everything still to discover.

The potential you sense in a new relationship is one of the exciting elements that can never be reintroduced. It is rather like anticipating your holiday on a paradise island by reading the brochure. While the holiday is in the future you can imagine it all to be perfect. The reality will be different. It might be very good indeed but it won't be paradise: you get sand in your picnic lunch, or painful sunburn, or your flight is delayed seven hours. Even if none of these things happen it *still* wouldn't be perfect or paradise: that's because you are a human being in a real location and life isn't like that.

In the same way, it is the *potential* of a relationship to be perfect – to be everything you could possibly wish for – that is exciting. Once the relationship is established you will experience the reality of it: very good, maybe, but not flawless; and neither are its future possibilities so completely unknown.

When you are in love the other person is partly a creation of your imagination, hopes and wishes. When you know the real person well you will have seen him or her laid low with a cold, sometimes irritable and contrary, depressed, or behaving in a way you find ridiculous, or any number of ordinary human failings alongside the good qualities. This knowledge can make you feel a range of emotions, some of them negative but many of them good: humour, pleasure, compassion, tolerance: the deeper, quieter aspects of love. 'Magic' and 'excitement' are inappropriate and feeling that they can be captured again is often destructive.

Many couples go on to find contentment and happiness together once the love has become 'real'. But some people, although they continue in the relationship – marrying, having children, building a life together – do so with a sense of disappointment. They don't put the necessary effort into the relationship to make it better because they feel that they shouldn't have to work to make a relationship good.

A smaller number of people chase the sensations of being in love forever. Some may never commit themselves to a relationship, but pass on to someone new whenever the feeling of being in love fades. Others may believe they can make a commitment, yet marry many times, thinking that falling in love with someone new is proof that their current marriage has gone wrong. Others may stay married to one person but have a series of affairs.

These people are either looking for that elusive love which will remain romantically heady forever or they are 'love addicts', junkies hooked on the sensations of first love, following the same pattern as alcoholics or drug addicts or even those exercise freaks who crave the 'joggers' endorphin high. They will have some thrills and fun but ultimate disappointment, especially if they believe in the myth that this is something that can last. The happiness of an altered state of consciousness brought on by love, drugs, drink or exercise can only be temporary. Love that is rooted in reality and that is worked on is the only kind that can bring genuine, lasting contentment.

This chapter has looked at love in general and some common attitudes towards it. Now we must consider how you can apply this to yourself and your own relationships.

2

IS THIS IT?

It is all very well to talk and think about love in theory. It is rather different when you are in love and trying to analyse your own feelings. This chapter is mainly for people who are newly in love and are deciding whether to make a serious commitment, although couples in long-term relationships might also find it useful.

As we saw in the first chapter, new love involves feelings so powerful and all-consuming that it is hard to think about them calmly and sensibly. Something only touched on in the last chapter was the sexual aspect of new love: sometimes it is the main element, and the difficulty is that strong lust can feel exactly the same as love.

This is not very helpful if you are in love and need to know how serious it is and whether you have found the person you should marry. How do you know whether what you are feeling is the 'real thing'? Does falling in love necessarily mean that you are compatible or that your relationship will work? This chapter attempts to help you answer these questions and looks at how you can spot potential problems (and sort them out) at this stage, using quizzes and tasks.

These quizzes are designed to make you think in a new way about your love. Their outcome can't predict your future happiness – you need a crystal ball for that. No one can guarantee that your relationship will be ideal or happy. The progress of a relationship involves many factors: how both of you develop and change and how major life events – from having children, to moving home, to your parents dying – affect you individually and as a couple and how you cope with the problems you encounter.

What the quizzes can do is show you things about yourself and your loved one *now*: what makes you both tick, where you think and feel alike and where you differ. Some of these similarities and differences are more important than others, but all should be thought about before you take the big step of settling down together. By reading this chapter, doing these quizzes and thinking hard about what it all means you are already giving yourself a better chance than most couples have. Relate counsellors are continually saddened by how many couples embark on the most important relationship of their lives knowing so little about each other's attitudes and expectations.

THE SECRET YOU

This doesn't mean that most couples rush into marriage without talking to each other. It is more complicated than that. The truth is that many people don't talk about their attitudes and expectations because *they don't know what they are*. This might sound like nonsense, but many of your most basic views on life have been developing since childhood without you thinking about them at all. Because they are a part of you, if ever you do think about them they seem so self-evident and true that you assume everyone else thinks the same way and that they are hardly worth mentioning. Some are so basic you may never put them into words, or they may be different from what you think you believe: they are a secret even from you.

Your early experiences of life in your family will be different in many ways from your loved one's. Some of those differences may be small, others more considerable, but they will result in differences of attitude that it might not occur to you to talk about.

It is because this process is so gradual and unconscious that it affects you in ways you have little knowledge of or control over. This is most obvious in people from cruel or unhappy backgrounds. As adults they might vow not to behave as their parents did but, mysteriously, they often find themselves doing and saying things that bear a marked similarity to their parents' actions and attitudes. The daughter who has suffered at the hands of an alcoholic father may find herself marrying an alcoholic husband, and her own children will suffer as she did. The thinking, conscious part of her mind hates the idea of an alcoholic, but 'something' makes her go for someone who has the potential to become one. That 'something' is what drives us all to be the people we are – it is the unconsciously learnt lessons of our upbringing. In our heads we may think it is wrong, but doing it somehow feels right.

One woman, a housewife and mother who had read extensively about feminism and believed in women's liberation, made great efforts to teach her son how he should behave in relationships and around the house. She could not understand why he grew up to have traditional attitudes towards his wife, home and children. The conscious part of his mind remembered her words, but she gave out an unspoken message every minute of his life in the way she behaved: waiting on his father and himself hand and foot, shaping in him a deep-down belief that this is how a woman should be. In contrast, the son of a working mother who felt neglected by her when he was young, always consciously chose women who were the complete opposite and who wanted to base their lives at home. After a while he picked fault with these women, found them boring and said he felt trapped, but he had no idea why this should be.

! ━━━━━━━━━━━━━ *Task* ━━━━━━━━━━━━━

Window on the past

Think about your parents' relationship and write short sentences to describe it under the following headings:

Love and affection
Did they kiss or show affection to each other in front of you? Were you aware of their sexual relationship?

Anger
Did they quarrel? How much? How did they do so? Did they shout, sulk, nag, hit out? If they never showed anger do you think they didn't feel it – or kept it in?

Housework
Who did what around the house?

Career
If either or both of your parents worked, how did they feel about their jobs or each other's? How did you feel about their work?

Crises
Were there any major happenings in their relationship, such as one of them having an affair? Redundancy? Bad reaction to bereavement in the family?

Parents
How did they treat you and your brothers or sisters? Did your mother treat you differently from the way your father did? How did they show you affection? How did they discipline you? Do you think they liked being parents?

Single parent
If you were brought up by a single parent was this because of death or divorce? Did your mother never marry your father? Was he unknown? Did your parent mind being single? Did your parent have other relationships? If your parents were divorced did you take sides? Did you see the absent parent? If one of your parents died how old were you and what do you remember of this? How did the parent you lived with talk about the other one?

There are no right answers to these questions. When you have written down your memories exchange lists with your partner and read what each other has to say and then discuss it. By understanding each other's family lives you will gain ideas about how and why you perhaps see marriage differently.

!

All of your ideas about men and women, husbands and wives, parents and children are built up in this way and will affect how you relate to your partner and the sort of life you want to make together.

One very straightforward example is provided by Liz and Matthew, who met as two junior executives in the same firm when they were in their twenties. Matthew fell in love with Liz for many reasons, including the fact that she was as good at her job as he was. When they married he was happy for Liz to go on working, and they even agreed that she would do so after she had children. But Matthew came from a family where the women did not go out to work. Soon after they were married Liz and Matthew started to have rows about the housework. The main burden of it always fell on Liz, and the 'help' Matthew gave was limited to the occasional washing-up or running a vacuum-cleaner over the carpet, after which he expected Liz to thank him and admire his handiwork. Consciously Matthew believed in equality, but his background had programmed him to assume that a woman would do all the 'looking after' in a relationship.

It's easy to see how this can happen, and much harder to see the same pattern in your own life or in your partner's. It does not mean you will necessarily repeat your parents' experiences, but you are much more likely to be able to construct the kind of life and relationship you think you want if you become aware of these unconscious expectations. Sometimes these expectations only surface much later in a relationship, if you have children, for example, and you become aware that you think your partner is behaving wrongly because of your in-built ideas of how a parent should behave. Or you may have vowed never to divorce because your parents' own divorce made you so unhappy, but somehow when it comes to a crisis point in your own relationship you take this option rather than working through it.

Because these ideas are below the surface of your mind, when you come to answer the quizzes about your expectations it is important to do so quickly and without much thought. What you need to do is write down your immediate reactions, not what you believe you *should* think.

But first let us get back to love.

THE REAL THING?

Love is a feeling, and for precisely this reason it is not easy to translate it into thought or words. The difficulty with your own feelings is that it is hard to see them objectively enough for you to explain or understand them well. When they are very strong, as when you fall in love, it is almost impossible.

When you are newly in love you may not even want to examine your feelings, but if you are thinking about getting married you will be wondering if you can trust the durability of what you are feeling.

Romantic love

There is no mistaking romantic love. Your heart really does beat faster. You can lose your appetite, get butterflies in your stomach, treat every telephone call with your loved one as an important event. It shows in the way you look: your skin glows, your eyes sparkle, you feel a constant current of energy and excitement. Everyone and everything else in your life momentarily reduces in importance. Nothing and no one is as interesting as the person who is making you feel like this.

But, as we saw in the first chapter, this highly-charged state leads to a distorted perception of your loved one and even of yourself. Until this stage passes your love has not left the world of fantasy. Your image of your loved one is so powerful that it is easy to ignore – or simply not see – the ordinary parts of his or her character that perhaps are disappointing or disturbing. In the same way, you yourself feel transformed by love. You want to be a better person – so you present yourself in the best possible light, hiding those parts you don't want the other to see. For these reasons there is a barrier between you, although it certainly doesn't feel like it.

Wanting your lover to be the perfect person of your fantasy can cause you to project qualities on to him or her that aren't actually there, very like the way a film is projected on to a blank screen.

Martin is a case in point. He came to Relate on his own because he was torn between his wife of five years and the woman with whom he had recently fallen in love. His story really started years before when he was eighteen and in love with Judith, a girl his own age. They were deeply in love, and as far as Martin was concerned Judith was perfect. But Martin felt that they were both too young to settle down. She was his first serious girlfriend and he thought he should play the field before committing himself. He duly played the field for two years, and at the end of the time was convinced that Judith was the girl for him. But when he looked her up again she was married to someone else. Within six months Martin too was married, to a girl he met on the rebound and who was the opposite of Judith in every way. They had two children and were moderately happy until Martin came across Samantha.

Samantha could have been Judith's sister. They looked very alike and had similar personalities. He fell for her immediately and they quickly started an affair. Martin loved his wife and his children but not in the way he loved Samantha. He felt guilty and torn, and hoped that counselling could help him sort himself out.

It was clear very quickly to the counsellor that as far as Martin was concerned Samantha *was* Judith – indeed Martin often called her Judith by mistake during the counselling sessions. Probing by the counsellor revealed in what respects they were different, but Martin couldn't see it – or didn't want to. He was so concerned to recreate the relationship he had had with Judith that he had projected all her qualities on to Samantha. The only problem he could see was the practical one of splitting up his family and hurting people he loved. Counselling couldn't progress because Martin was unable to face reality.

Romance and reality

The romantic stage is usually a time of courting – you send each other love notes and have long, loving phone calls. You buy each other little presents; he brings flowers, chocolates or other symbols of love.

To many people these romantic gestures 'mean' love. They are the visible proof that you are loved and when they go some people feel that love has gone too. This is not, of course, the case, but it can cause trouble when the relationship is progressing to another level, particularly if the courting stops abruptly with marriage.

At some point ordinary sensible thinking must take over so that you can sort out the depth and reality of your feelings. Being sensible is the last thing you want to be when caught up in the sheer pleasure of being in love. As one counsellor says, you should enjoy the feelings as long as they last – so long as you are aware that they can't last. Another counsellor points out that having a romantic time together to look back on gives you the will to cope with the bad times when they come.

Problems come when you indulge in this essentially unrealistic state and are reluctant to see the real person beyond the fantasy you have developed. One woman who had married a 'pillar of strength' could not bear him to show any vulnerability – consequently in years to come, when she was more able to cope, he was unable to share his deepest feelings with her. Counsellors say that some people can be just as blind twenty years into a marriage as they were when they first fell in love, and this has allowed them to live with their partners while never truly knowing them, causing problems to build up over the years. That is why it is important to put the happy, positive feelings to good use and find out as much as you can about each other at this early stage of the relationship.

Romantic love will not tell you whether you are essentially right for each other, which is a more complex issue. There is no foolproof way of telling this but the section and the quizzes on compatibility further on will help.

?_____ **Quiz** _____

About the house

These are some of the regular things that are involved in living together as a family. Who should do them? Against each item write M (if it should be him) F (if it should be her) or B (if it should be both partners). Both write what you think and discuss any differences of opinion.

Drawing up shopping lists

Cooking

Hoovering

Washing floors

Cleaning the toilet

Cleaning the fridge

Polishing

Doing the washing

Washing/cleaning major items
(curtains, blankets etc)

Paying household bills

Heavy gardening work

Dealing with plumbing/electrics

Choosing the car

Household budgeting

Decorating decisions

Wallpapering

Washing baby's nappies

Shopping

Washing up

Sweeping floors

Cleaning the bathroom

Spring-cleaning cupboards

Dusting

Sorting washing loads

Ironing

Mending clothes

Making clothes

Putting up shelves

Planning the garden

Clearing gutters

Maintaining the car

Cleaning the windows

Painting

Changing the baby's nappy

Choosing baby's clothes

_____ **?**

_____ LOVE AND EXPERIENCE _____

Your own experiences of falling in love are also important in determining how realistic or lasting your feelings are.

Of course this means it is most difficult to assess your feelings when you fall in love for the first time. Teenagers who fall passionately in love are rightly annoyed when they are told that it is not the real thing. What they are feeling is perfectly real and may be even stronger for being the first time. Usually it doesn't last long – it can be over in a matter of days or weeks. In retrospect they themselves are as likely as anyone else to dismiss it as 'not really love'.

Teenagers often find it hard to remember what it was they saw in the first love – or the first few – as their tastes change and mature so fast. Many young people find that part of the intoxication they feel is the pleasure and excitement of being loved. Finding that someone thinks you're wonderful and is in love with you makes you feel gloriously special – powerful at any time, and particularly when you are young. Some people go on to marry their first love, or their first serious love, while they are in their teens or early twenties and still in the long process of growing up. Some of these relationships last, but many break up as they find that within a few years they have turned into very different people.

Each time you fall in love you have a better sense of how reasonably rooted the feeling is. Your own experience shows you that the marvellously heady feelings we described before don't last, and as you mature and your experience of people widens you also become more choosy. You know yourself better and are more likely to be aware whether what you are feeling is only a passing physical attraction. Falling in love when you are more settled in yourself and your way of life means that your choices are likely to be more realistic.

Relate counsellors find that couples who marry from their late twenties onwards have a better chance of making a go of it. If you have had more than one serious relationship you have a better sense of what works for you. Between the ages of twenty and thirty your needs and interests are going to change and develop. Knowing whether you have met the right partner comes with knowing yourself.

If you are young and in love this might make you impatient. Is age that important? If you have found the person you want to marry now is it bound to go wrong? Of course not. There is no magical right age to marry. Very young marriages are statistically more *likely* to go wrong, but you are individuals, not statistics. Maturity doesn't necessarily bring wisdom or self-knowledge and, as we saw in the first chapter, falling in love disastrously can happen at any age. What is far more important is your essential compatibility and your desire to make it work.

! ——————————— *Task* ———————————

Associations

Write a list of anyone your partner reminds you of – family, friend, old flame, famous person – in looks, behaviour or any other way.

Talk together about your lists and what you feel about these other people.

!

THE TEST OF TIME

Making a big decision when you are madly in love is risky when you remember how similar it is to being under the influence of drink or drugs. It is sensible to give your love a chance to prove itself before you set the wedding day.

Knowing how long to give it can be a problem in itself. When you are very much in love it is hard to imagine your feelings will ever change; strong feelings of being 'in love' can last for around two years. When it lasts as long as this you can be forgiven for thinking that it can go on forever, but this is still not so. The 'hangover' always comes, though if you have been building a worthwhile relationship in the meantime it might not be so disturbing.

Even counsellors are divided about how long you should wait before marrying. Some believe that if you marry before the 'in love' feelings have changed you are more committed to weathering the bad times of the hangover period. Others believe that you should wait until you have gone through this time and shown each other that there are firmer foundations to your love. But all counsellors agree that it is essential for you to have withstood the test of how you handle problems between the two of you before you make a life commitment.

An example of a couple who thought they had tested their relationship but had, in fact, avoided problems is Vanessa and Bill. Bill was a married man, and his affair with Vanessa had lasted six good years. Their 'in love' feelings had lasted throughout this period, fed by the fact that they could only snatch time together – time in which they concentrated fully on each other as lovers do in the early part of a relationship. They finally agreed that he should leave his wife and marry Vanessa.

They had had problems in the course of their affair. Vanessa had wanted Bill to leave his wife soon after they met, and sometimes they would argue about that. Occasionally Bill would become very jealous over Vanessa's friendships with other men and even her girlfriends, which would cause friction between them. But their pattern when they argued was to have a cooling-off period. They would not see or speak to each for a few days until the angry feelings had faded. Then one of them would phone and apologise or make a joke of it and they would be back to their usual loving selves.

The turbulent time of Bill's divorce and when he moved in with Vanessa nearly broke them up. It was distressing for both of them, and made them tense and irritable with each other. Previously they had seen each other at their best, now both were too fraught to be at anything but their worst.

They immediately discovered that they had developed no useful way of dealing with the problems that arose between them. Living together made it impossible for them to operate the cooling-off system, so the anger didn't fade. Rows either continued or turned into a war of sulks. Their relationship deteriorated until they were terrified that it had all been a disastrous mistake. Their fantasy love was being tested by reality in the most brutal way.

In their case counselling was able to allow them to uncover the good feelings they still had about each other and help them to deal with negative feelings more usefully. They did go on to marry and although their relationship was never as idyllic as they imagined it would be when they were having the affair, it was good.

Similar problems affect couples who marry before they have hit any difficulties together – which are dealt with in the chapter Who Are You Marrying? about the problems that can arise during the first year of marriage.

Meeting problems destroys some of the euphoria of being in love, and allows you to see beyond it to whether there are aspects that are longer lasting than euphoria and passion – and more reliable. These include interests and goals that you share, and an agreement about how you both see your future roles.

Love is made up of many elements, which can form a good backbone to a relationship and help to make it last.

THE BACKBONE OF LOVE

Of the elements that make up love, some are more enduring than others – it is natural, for instance, for sexual passion to become less strong as the years pass. Other aspects are more reliable, in that they can become stronger with the years:

• **Liking.** How much do you actually like your partner? Like can seem a rather weedy emotion compared to love, but it is one of the most important components in making your relationship last. It might seem surprising, but some people fall in love and form relationships with partners they don't like very much. If you enjoy each other's company, find each other interesting as human beings, approve of the way each other thinks and behaves, you stand a good chance of feeling the same once the 'in love' feelings have passed. If there are things that irritate or bore you about your partner, or of which you disapprove, or which make you feel cross or contemptuous, these will matter to you more once you have stopped feeling madly in love. A question to ask yourself is, 'Would I want to be friends with this person if we weren't in love?'

❛━━━━━━━━━ Talking point ━━━━━━━━━

Love is . . .

Spend half an hour talking about love together. For five minutes
one of you describe why you love the other; then it is the other's
turn. After this, take it in turns to describe for five minutes what a
loving married relationship will be like. For the last ten minutes
discuss what you have both said.

If you don't want to do this ask yourself why. If it is difficult
talking about such good things, won't it be even harder to talk about
problems?

❜

● **Humour.** Being able to laugh together and sharing a sense of humour
is also important in helping love to last. But humour has another function.
Humour makes for tolerance. It means being able to approach the
smaller obstacles in your relationship with a sense of proportion, not
making a mountain out of a molehill or taking minor problems too
seriously.

● **Respect.** This old-fashioned concept has a vital part to play in
keeping love alive. It means not treating your partner with more
rudeness and less thought than you would a friend or acquaintance. The
phrase 'Love means never having to say you're sorry' has a lot to answer
for. You *should* say you're sorry if you have done something you feel bad
about. Saying thoughtless, hurtful, unkind things to loved ones is quite
common. (Phrases such as, 'You look awful in that', 'You're so bloody
stupid', 'I can't stand the sound of your voice any longer' and hundreds
more.) The rule should be: would I talk to anyone else like this? If the
answer is no, think twice before you do. If something is upsetting you,
finding a nicer way to put it often gets the results you want.

Respect also means you are prepared to listen to each other: the
ability to listen being one of the secrets of enduring love.

● **Generosity.** Generous feelings towards your loved one are part of
'true' love. 'In love' feelings are usually selfish. 'In love' means wanting
things for yourself: your lover close to you, behaving in ways that make
you happy. Genuinely wanting something purely for the good of your
partner is a very different matter, especially when there is no real benefit
to yourself. For instance, if your partner wants to develop a hobby which
means you have less time together than you would like, your generous

feelings mean you encourage it with pleasure. It means allowing your partner to be an individual with needs that occasionally clash with yours. Being able to give each other 'space' is a positive move forwards from the complete togetherness of first love, which does not allow for individual growth and change. The fact that you can find happiness and pleasure apart is one of the first shocks in a developing relationship, but allowing it to happen adds to love.

• **Effort.** This last element is perhaps the most important – the X ingredient of lasting love. Putting effort into love even while it is good builds it up for the future. Making the necessary effort when things go wrong is essential if your relationship is going to survive problems and become still better, as was shown by Alison and Mike in the last chapter. This is dealt with in more detail in the chapter on Change, Problems and Crises. It is also the main message of this book: being prepared for problems to happen and being willing to negotiate them together says even more for your chances of living happily and lovingly together than how strongly you love or like each other at the beginning.

How much of the good feelings of love remain also depends quite heavily on how compatible you are.

COMPATIBILITY

Being compatible means that you naturally tend to get on with each other. The most important elements include sharing basic aims, the same feelings about what you want out of a relationship, and how you foresee family life and your own roles within it.

What makes you compatible?

Certain obvious factors in your background help with compatibility. If you come from a family of the same or similar race, religion, size and social class, have had similar educations and are around the same age you are more *likely* to have the kinds of things in common that ensure durability in a relationship. These factors are particularly powerful when you decide to marry and other people – particularly your family and friends – feel it is their right to tell you what they think about the decision . This is looked at again in the next chapter, Who Are You Marrying?

But if this were a strict rule, only people who married the boy or girl next door would go on to have happy marriages. 'Next door' marriages break up too, and marriages where there are great differences can thrive.

More important are the values and ideas you have developed about life, love and relationships, which the quizzes, tasks and talking points are designed to make obvious to you. An unhappy childhood, for instance can make you expect quite different things than would a partner who had happy experiences, even if you appear to come from identical backgrounds.

This doesn't mean you should ignore important differences in age, religion, race and all the other aspects. They can make for difficulties if you pretend they don't exist – perhaps not now while you are very much in love – but later when the relationship settles down, you are building a network of friendships together, and if you decide to have children. Being aware of the possible problems they can cause is only sensible and means you are ready to cope with whatever comes.

What will happen if you are not compatible?

If there are significant differences in your experiences, or you find that you think quite differently on important, fundamental matters, then areas where you clash, or things that will make you unhappy, are likely to crop up early in your relationship.

Matters such as disagreements over when to have a baby – or whether to have one at all – can give you trouble early on if you haven't talked them through and reached acceptable compromises. Problems may also emerge one by one over the years as differences are highlighted by events in your lives.

This happens to essentially compatible couples too, as they also change and develop as the years pass. Any emerging differences have to be dealt with and negotiated.

By identifying areas where you are out of step with each other you can start to deal with potential problems before they grow out of hand.

! ——————————— *Task* ———————————

Role swap

Put yourself in your partner's shoes and describe yourself through his or her eyes. Pick on points you think your partner finds irritating or would like to change about you.

Discuss together whether you have got it right. !

The attraction of opposites

It is a commonplace that opposites attract. What has this to do with compatibility? Relate counsellors refer to this as the 'marital fit' – where two people who are unalike fit together like jigsaw pieces, each giving the other something they lack.

A 'good fit' might be between a jolly, outgoing, frivolous person who teams up with someone who is shy and quiet – but steady and reliable. When it works they harmonise with each other. The fit works especially well if they are compatible in other ways: for instance, the man is the solid steady one and the woman more lively and emotional and they both believe that this is the right way for men and women to behave; he quietly providing the means for the family while she deals with the sociable and emotional aspects of the home.

Trouble can start when one or other changes for some reason. Confidence built up over the years can make him more extrovert, or some unhappiness may make her less bubbly or more moody. The fit is not as exact any more, and this leads to tension. In a good and flexible relationship the couple comes to terms with this and is able to adjust.

Some couples, however, fit together in a way that is very tight but not so healthy. To become a full and effective human being someone may need to develop coping skills, but instead he or she marries a person who does all the coping for them both. The 'coper' is frightened of losing control, and rather than facing that fear and loosening up chooses to be with a partner in a situation that means not having to try. This kind of fit stops each of them developing fully and can lead to an unhealthy dependency of which they are both frightened to let go. In many cases they dislike or resent their partners for the very reasons they chose them. For example, the fearful person, afraid to cope alone, can find the other too controlling and restricting. If circumstances force a change on either of them the relationship can fall apart because they have no idea how to manage without the fit.

Does compatibility now mean happiness later?

Compatibility gives you a head start, but changes in your situation and yourself can throw up unforeseen differences between you. Nothing stays the same – which is exciting as well as disturbing. As we have said before, being prepared for change, being flexible and ready to make the effort for your relationship is then what counts.

_____ LIVING TOGETHER _____

Nowadays it is not uncommon for a couple who are in love to move in together. Living together can be a stepping-stone to marriage, a trial marriage or even just like marriage. It can also be a different kind of relationship that doesn't turn into anything else and eventually ends when it no longer suits one or both of you.

But for those who see it as a trial marriage or a stepping-stone to marriage, or a test of compatibility, it is important to look at whether it can effectively be any of these things. Will it tell you better than anything else whether you are right for each other?

Living together is more acceptable than it was, though still not entirely so. Some parents think it is fine for other people's children but not their own, others feel it is all right for their sons but not for their daughters. To many minds it is still a relatively unconventional step. For these reasons most people have less clear ideas about what kind of relationship it is and less defined expectations about the roles of each partner within it.

One counsellor notices that clients of hers who have lived together seem to divide daily tasks more evenly between them – there are less obviously 'women's' and 'men's' jobs. She also finds that after marriage the men in these relationships seem more able to talk about their feelings (something most men find hard to do). She thinks that it is because the option of living together attracts less conventional men who would be less inclined to worry about a 'non-macho' display of feelings.

Why live together rather than marry?

People move in together for a number of different reasons. When sex outside marriage was taboo there was no such option and many married out of sheer physical attraction. Now some people acknowledge that their love is passionate and powerful but don't know how lasting it is. They want to make the right decision and marry at the right moment. Living together can be a time to test whether it is a temporary euphoria, sexually produced, or real love. Others don't think about it much but want to move in together because the attraction between them is so powerful that they don't see any good reason to wait.

Some couples regard it quite clearly as a trial marriage to see how they suit, or as a logical halfway step in a relationship, like being engaged. Others live together because although they love each other they might feel too young or in other ways not ready to make any final decisions about settling down. Still others make the move because it's the done thing in their set and they 'might as well'.

Marriage is a definite commitment, while living together is more of a trial – a time for thinking, 'Do we really want this commitment?'

The difficulty is that one of you might make the decision for a reason that turns out to be different from your partner's. For example, one of you may believe it is a stepping stone to marriage, while the other has assumed that it is purely for sexual and convenience reasons.

How good a test of compatibility is it?

It might seem obvious that living together before marriage will show you whether you will be compatible when married, but this isn't necessarily so. It certainly highlights immediate, practical issues to do with sharing a life: how much you like each other, how you deal with disagreements, the question of money, who cooks, cleans, shops, remembers the milk on the way home from work. If you have very different ideas about this, you're going to clash.

What living together won't automatically do is tell you about your hidden expectations of marriage. Because your expectations are part of the 'secret you' you might not even be aware that you will expect things to be different once you do marry. Counsellors have noted that couples who have lived together for years can have talked as little about what they want when they marry as those who marry after a whirlwind romance. They assume that because they are living together that they must want the same things from life.

❛————————— Talking point ═══════

Marriage is . . .

These are four statements made by different people about what they think marriage is.

'A declaration to the world that you love each other and plan to stay together forever.'
'The best kind of relationship in which to bring up children.'
'A relationship within which it is possible to work through the bad times together, so that the bond between you is strengthened.'
'For people who are in love, and should be dissolved when they are no longer in love.'

Discuss together what you think of these statements. Can you formulate a statement of your own?

❜

How different is it from marriage?

Can a marriage certificate really make that much difference to the way you behave towards each other? It shouldn't, but in practice it does – if your ideas about how married life should be are different from the life you have constructed while living together.

When Karen and Alex were living together they shared chores and made the effort to do things together. Every week they had a special night out – they went out for a meal or to the cinema or theatre. Alex was the one who was most keen to marry. He was longing to have a proper home, a legal wife and children – like most of his friends and colleagues. Karen was reluctant to stop working and have children. But she loved Alex and finally agreed to marry him, give up her job and start a family.

Karen thought she was prepared for the changes this would mean in her life – but she wasn't prepared for the way Alex changed. The first thing to go was the special night out. Alex began to treat her in quite a different way and abruptly stopped doing anything around the house. Karen had imagined that their relationship would go on in the same way as when they were living together; Alex saw it as something else completely. She was angry, he was bewildered: they had not thought any of it through.

In contrast, when James and Geraldine married they were both keen to do so having had a wonderful two years of living together. They were a very good-looking couple who had fallen in love on first meeting and moved in together quite quickly.

The two years of living together were great fun. Geraldine remembers that setting up home was like playing with a doll's house. James said, 'When we were living together she was exciting, she had a good job and we had lots of laughs.' Eventually, however, they decided it was time to start a family and they got married. They had two children, and eight years later were divorcing.

Geraldine had had a very unhappy childhood, with a violent alcoholic father who would disappear for weeks on end. She wanted home life for her own children to be perfect and for James to be the model father. As soon as they were married Geraldine plunged into domesticity. She gave up her job and began to put pressure on James to become the husband and father she wanted him to be. He had to be home on the dot every day and do his duty by her and the children. The fun-loving Geraldine disappeared and she became demanding and hysterical, threatening to commit suicide when James made it clear that he was more keen on putting effort into his developing career than into his increasingly restrictive family life.

For James marriage meant fun and togetherness with the woman he loved – but she had seemed to disappear after the wedding. For Geraldine marriage meant a happy family on her terms, but by forcing her own vision on James she got the opposite.

These experiences are common: hidden expectations about how a husband or wife should behave often don't surface until you are married.

The decision to marry

On average there is a make-or-break two-year boundary. Many couples either decide to marry after two years or split up. For couples who see living together as a stepping stone to marriage, two years seems a decent interval. Many say, 'Well, we're still together and it obviously works so we might as well get married.'

Of course this varies and some people go on to marry after living together much longer than two years. It is most often the decision to have children or when the woman finds she's pregnant that decides the matter. One counsellor remarked that, 'With couples I've seen, the longer they have lived together the harder they find it to make the decision to get married.'

Unfortunately some couples make the decision to marry when all is *not* good between them. They think, 'We're not getting on terribly well, but maybe if we marry it will improve.' Or else they marry because of outside pressures from family and friends, who keep asking 'When is it going to be?'

After marriage

As we have seen, the relationship can change after marriage as the couple begin to live out their own ideas about the behaviour of husbands and wives and parents. But there are other factors that can bring about change too.

• **Loss of freedom.** While you are living together your options are still open. Many people find it difficult to adjust to the fact that they have made a choice that removes these other options. One half of the couple might feel more secure because of this while the other feels trapped.

• **The shifting balance.** In some relationships one half of the couple is much keener on marriage than the other. That person can, unconsciously, be on his or her best behaviour before marriage – and then feel able to relax after the wedding day. There is a balance of power when one is holding off marrying which automatically shifts after the ceremony and can make the relationship feel very different.

- **Sex and romance.** A couple who are living together often continue to behave romantically towards each other, treating it as a courting stage. This usually goes after a period of marriage, when it might be missed by one of them.

Sex often becomes more routine. Many couples who arrive in counselling after some years of marriage look back on their living together days as particularly passionate. Sex in marriage seems dull and ordinary in comparison.

This can be explained partly by the fact that many tend to marry after about two years, when the 'in love' feelings are passing and when passion also tends to wane. But others stop trying in their sex lives, sometimes because of their subconscious belief that marital sex should not be inventive. Other reasons for sex becoming disappointing are dealt with in the chapter on Sex.

There are others for whom sex becomes better after marriage – usually those who have felt guilty about sex outside marriage.

- **Money.** A couple who are living together will often keep separate bank accounts. When they marry they pool their incomes and the woman may give up her job. This can cause stress and produce new problems that neither have talked about.

! ══════════ *Task* ══════════

I should . . . you should . . .

Take a large sheet of paper each and divide into four sections. On each page write these headings for the sections:

A husband should . . .
A wife should . . .
A mother should . . .
A father should . . .

Without pausing to think too much, or discussing it, both of you fill in these sections on your separate pieces of paper with whatever comes into your mind about how a husband/wife/mother/father should behave towards their partners and children. You can also put in any 'shouldn'ts' that come to mind. When you have finished, swap sheets of paper and talk about what you have both written.

!

When you live together for years

Some couples live together for many years, not marrying, but in every other way behaving like a married couple. These couples have made a commitment to each other in their own way and feel as good as married.

In a few cases it is because they are aware of the negative expectations they have developed about marriage and are frightened of repeating bad experiences from their childhood in their own lives. One counsellor saw a couple who were going through a crisis and she discovered that they had never married (this was not the cause of the problem). Tina's parents had argued violently throughout their marriage and part of her assumed that marriage meant strife. She wouldn't marry Mark even after their child was born, though she changed her surname to his.

Sometimes knowing that your options are technically open keeps the relationship good because you are more likely to work through problems rather than ignore them.

Dealing with problems

All relationships go through changes – it is not unique to people who have lived together first. One counsellor notices that couples who have lived together first tend to come for counselling earlier in their relationship than those who married straight away: typically after about seven years rather than the average fourteen. She says that their problems are no worse than anybody else's, but they seem to want to sort them out at an earlier stage than those who have never lived together.

It appears that they are more likely to acknowledge a problem than the other couples, who wait until it becomes acute. Most of them had also tried to do something about the problems before coming for counselling. In her experience couples who marry in the conventional way seem more likely to bury disappointments and unfulfilled expectations until the problem becomes too big to ignore.

This counsellor's experience seems to suggest that people who have lived together are more cautious about relationships and less likely to believe that falling in love should conquer all.

Crises and living together

If you are living with someone now and a serious problem has arisen in your relationship you will be wondering if you should ever marry. Dealing with problems together is no different because you are not yet married, so you will find that most of your questions will be answered in the chapter on Change, Problems and Crises.

?_____**Quiz**_____

It's important to me

This quiz is in three sections. In the first two number the points in what you consider to be their order of importance. You can copy it so that you both do this separately without knowing what the other has put.

What I want from a relationship
a) to find my 'other half'; b) not to be lonely; c) to find someone to have children with; d) to be loved; e) to be in love and passionate forever; f) to be looked after; g) to have someone to look after; h) to have a good sexual relationship; i) to build a home; j) to have a lifelong friend; k) something else (write what it is) .

What I think is important in life
a) a loving relationship; b) a career; c) money; d) the environment; e) education; f) religion; g) bringing up my children; h) travel; i) hobbies and interests; j) politics; k) something else (write what it is)

I get angry about
(in this case pick your top five)
stupidity; cruelty to children/old people; rape or violence to women; environmental destruction; racial issues; political issues; lack of money; lack of freedom; being told what to do; feminism; male chauvinism; being criticised; rudeness; terrorism; cheating on marriage partner; being lied to; being ignored; being treated coldly; someone being angry with me;

Look at what you have both chosen and discuss your choices when you have finished.

_____**?**

3

WHO ARE YOU MARRYING?

You are marrying the person you love best in the world. Your wedding should be the happiest day of your life, and your honeymoon – your first real time alone together as husband and wife – should be the holiday of a lifetime.

All of this can be true, but it isn't always. From a purely practical point of view, the organisation involved in getting married is a tiring, stressful business and stress does not produce the light-hearted feelings of happiness. And the practical aspects of the wedding are not the only ones that cause stress. Other factors in the build-up to the wedding and the honeymoon can also stop this from being a happy time.

This chapter concentrates on the difficulties of this period and the first year or so after marriage. That is not to say that it will all be relevant to you – your own wedding and the aftermath might be as blissful as you hope – but if you do hit one or more of these problems it is as well to know that you are not alone. For the many couples who do find this a worrying or problematic time, guilt at not being happy is an added burden and they tend to ignore problems that crop up at this stage, terrified that looking hard at them will reveal that the decision to marry was a mistake. By knowing that mixed feelings and other problems are normal you are better able to see them for what they are and tackle them immediately.

WHO ARE YOU MARRYING?

The reason for the rather odd title to this chapter is, as we have seen, that you can fall in love and agree to marry someone without really knowing him or her very well.

It also refers to the fact that except in very rare instances the person you are marrying is not alone in the world. Your loved one is part of a package which includes family and friends. It is possible to ignore this fact when you are courting and wrapped up in each other to the exclusion of everyone else, but during the run-up to the wedding, and after you are married, you will learn to what extent you are marrying into each other's families and networks of friendships.

The family

Your family is the single most important element in making you the person you have become. Love the members of your family or hate them, they have had a great influence on you. One of the best ways of understanding yourself and your partner is to look back on childhood experiences and how the members of your family related to one another. If you haven't yet done the Window on the Past task in the previous chapter, it is worth doing so now.

The decision to marry brings with it the active involvement of your families, however distant you have become from them. You will hear their views and strongly expressed pleasure or displeasure and they will want to meet and get to know your intended – who is having the same experience with his or her family. With all the different people and opinions involved it would be great good fortune if everyone loved everyone else, and it is quite common for one or both of you to feel rather uncomfortable during this period.

Family approval

It is at this time that difficulties to do with nonstandard marriages are most evident. By this we mean marriages where there are important differences in age, social class, race, religion, education and so on. Families can feel it is their right to come out and say if they don't approve, and some do everything in their power to stop a marriage going ahead if they think it is going to be a disaster.

This throws up strong emotions, particularly in you, the people who are about to marry. Yet it is at this time that you need to be most cool and sensible about what you are doing. If you don't get on with your family you must be sure that you are not marrying to get back at them. Your decision to marry must be based only on the good relationship between the two of you. One counsellor saw a couple who were having sexual difficulties early in their marriage. She counselled them for several months, during which time it was revealed that they had married with a spirit of defiance because her parents thought he wasn't good enough for her. The fact that the parents disapproved had added spice to their sex life, but when the pleasure of outwitting the parents had faded so did the sexual bond and they found they had little to say to each other and still less in common.

If you are fond of your family and care what they think, then their displeasure at your decision will worry you. This is another good reason for examining the true basis of your relationship. Loving families will usually come round in the end if they see you are happy.

You should also look out for parental pressure the other way – sometimes families are so eager to see you married off that they will push you towards a wedding before you yourself are sure that it is right.

Occasionally families also disapprove of apparently perfectly well-matched people: it is hard for loving fathers and mothers to think anyone is good enough for their sons and daughters. Whatever the reason, family disapproval or pressure causes you to explain your decision to marry and to do that you have to be sure in your own mind about what you are doing. Acknowledging and dealing with problems at this stage saves greater problems later.

?——————————**Quiz**——————————

The wedding

These are some of the elements that make up a wedding. Give each one marks out of five to show how important you think it is.

1 = not important at all
2 = OK, but could do without it
3 = quite important
4 = very important
5 = essential

Our vows to each other	Promising to obey
The service	The music at the ceremony
A beautiful dress	Bridesmaids/pages
The best man	All my family being there
All my friends being there	The cake
Champagne/range of drinks	Lovely food
Music/entertainment at the party	A good photographer
Having a video made	Getting in the local paper
Groom in morning dress/smart new clothes	Confetti
	The best man's speeches
The father's/other relative's speeches	New 'going away' clothes
Expensive presents	Expensive invitations
Being the centre of attention	A good stag/hen night

Compare your feelings on these elements and discuss the ones about which you think most differently.

——————————————————————————**?**

Family closeness

How much your respective families will matter in your relationship is
dependent partly on how close you feel to them. If one of you comes from
a close family with whom you want to retain constant contact, then that
family is going to remain an element within your marriage. If both of you
are close to your families it follows that both families will be of some
importance. This can be a good and positive thing, enriching your
marriage and offering any children you might have the security of a large
extended family. But the more people who are involved the more the
chances of friction are increased, especially during the early stages.

Whether or not you are close to your family you are likely to be
sensitive about them. You don't like to hear your parents or brothers and
sisters criticised even if you are critical of them yourself. Your partner
will feel the same. It does not follow that because you love someone you
will necessarily like or love the members of their family to whom they
feel attached. Sometimes your partner feeling strong love for someone
else can make you feel jealous and resentful, even if it is a member of
the family.

The important point to bear in mind is that in the period around a
wedding families will be much more central and active than they will be
later on. As time goes on they will usually settle more into the background
of your life. Equally you must be aware that families do not go away.
You will have to find an acceptable way of coming to terms with them
so that your married life will not be affected by bad feelings. That
depends, as most marital issues do, on sensitive co-operation between
the two of you. That is, respecting each other's feelings about the matter
and negotiating compromises.

Janet and Matthew are an example of a couple whose marriage was
affected by the influence of one family – in this case Janet's. They had
lived together happily for eighteen months when Matthew proposed.
Their home had been a rather squalid rented flat in the centre of town.
Both of them worked and every Saturday Matthew played football and
Janet would accompany him and his mates to a spit-and-sawdust pub
after the match. Janet was keen to marry and as Matthew was happy
with their life together he thought they might as well.

Immediately after Matthew proposed Janet's mother swooped down
on them. She was paying for and organising the wedding so she was
always in and out, talking about the arrangements. Her plans, however,
stretched further than the day itself. Soon after they decided to marry
she began to criticise the flat: 'You can't stay here after you're married,
of course,' she would say. She began house hunting for them and found
a place near where she and Janet's father lived, in a nicer, more middle-
class part of town. Janet began talking about giving up work.

Although all this made Matthew understandably nervous he didn't talk about his fears. He concentrated on the good relationship he had with Janet and the pleasant life they had together. But after they married everything deteriorated.

Janet gave up work and started to talk about having children. She stopped being happy about Matthew playing football, and didn't want to spend Saturday nights with his friends down the pub any more. In counselling she admitted that she had previously put up with this purely for Matthew's sake and because she wanted to marry him. She assumed he would change after marriage. He had thought marriage would include all the good elements of living together, with time for his mates plus the perks of two incomes. He was not ready to think about starting a family. These were serious differences of expectations which many other couples have to face, but matters were made worse by Janet's family.

Married life threw them together with her family, which had not been the case when they lived together. They were expected to visit them every weekend and often during the week. Matthew couldn't stand his in-laws and found their values suffocating. He said that all they thought about was 'a nice home and a mortgage.' As far as he was concerned, life was about spending your money as you got it and having a good time.

Matthew soon felt trapped by Janet's family. He started to drink more heavily and stay out with his mates. He used the excuse of working late to avoid Janet and her family. During the counselling they were unable to find common ground and they decided to separate. They were at different life stages: he still wanted to be one of the lads and she needed to settle down. The close involvement of her family didn't help, though it should be said that if their expectations had matched this probably wouldn't have been such a problem.

!————————————— *Task* —————————————

My other life

Make two lists, one of all the family members you see regularly, the other including all your friends. Next to each person's name write how often you would like to see them after you are married.

D = daily
W = weekly
M = monthly
O = occasionally
F = Festivals – Christmas, birthdays etc
N = never
    Compare lists with your partner.

!

Your friends

Relationships with each other's friends also have an impact on you during this time, though not to quite the degree that families have.

If you are marrying young you may well have come from the same group of friends, but the later you meet the more likely you are to have very different sets of friends – relationships sometimes stretching right back to early childhood.

The stronger your friendships the more they will matter in your life together, at least in the early days. Good, long-standing friends will have as much to say about your marriage as your family – and in some cases you might value their opinions more highly than you do your family's.

Again there is more chance of a problem if your relationship is nonstandard in any way. The bigger the gap between you and your loved one, the bigger the potential gap between your loved one and your friends – and between you and his or her friends. The main problem Roger and Amy encountered, for example, was their friends. Amy was twelve years older than Roger, who was twenty-four. She found she had little in common with many of Roger's male friends, who were less mature than he was, and she felt very uncomfortable with their girlfriends, most of whom were in their early twenties, with one or two in their teens. Roger, for his part, felt awkward with Amy's sophisticated friends, especially with the men who were established in their careers and approaching middle age.

Jealousy in friendships can cause difficulties. Best friends can feel pushed out by your new lover – and your lover can feel resentful of people who have known you so much longer and better than he or she has. Friends who feel like this can magnify any problems that do arise between you and your partner by taking your side and coming between you during bad times.

After marriage friendships tend to change – if not at first, then slowly as time goes on. Social habits can make for some problems between you if, like Matthew, you want to continue the same pattern of behaviour with your friends after you are married. Most couples come to a compromise about their earlier friendships; some naturally drop away, others are weeded out. You mix more with those of each other's friends you do like and make new friendships together. This is natural. As your circumstances change you usually feel drawn to people having similar experiences – for instance, if you have children you find yourself more interested in couples who are at the same stage.

Nevertheless friendships can be the cause of stress during these pre-wedding days and it is useful to keep a sense of proportion about them.

WEDDING PREPARATIONS

The organisation of a big event is stressful. A wedding is even more stressful than most because it is such an important social and life-changing occasion. Everyone feels emotional, not just the bride and groom but family and friends as well. All are aware that it is a big step – that your future and your happiness are involved in this decision.

Many couples decide to have the biggest and best wedding they can afford. They want it to be a wonderful day to look back on – but it is important to be aware of how much it can also take out of you. These are some of the points to think about:

● **Money.** A proper white wedding, with all the trimmings and a big reception, represents a major expenditure. This fact is important to many families as well as to the couple involved. Some parents save for years so that they can give a daughter a 'good send off' when the time comes. Knowing that you or your family have spent such large sums of money is an added pressure at this time, especially if you feel the money could have been used elsewhere.

Many people spend more than perhaps they should. There is often a feeling that if you don't go for the most expensive options then you are also skimping on your emotional investment: the amount of money equals the amount of love. Pressure comes from wanting to do as well as or better than other friends and family: the best photographer, the best video firm, the best caterers.

● **Organisation.** One counsellor describes the wedding preparations as a machine that starts from the time the couple set the date. Once started, the machine appears to become unstoppable, which is in itself nerve-wracking.

Very often one person takes charge of most of the organising, usually still the bride's mother. Both families become very involved at this stage and it can highlight potential difficulties for the future.

Sometimes the organisation is taken completely out of your hands by whoever is paying for it. Some couples don't feel they are involved enough, which can only add to the impression that the unstoppable machine is bearing you along whether you want it to or not, as well as making you feel that any doubts about marrying are not allowed.

Guest lists involve friction too. Whom, among members of each family, should be invited – or left out – and which friends are to be included? It is always difficult to know who to invite to any party, never mind the most important party of your life. It also makes you aware of who is important to your partner and why. This is a test of your negotiating skills when you are not at your most calm.

• **Your emotions.** Underlying all these potential problems is the fact that you are making a major decision. Few people go into marriage thinking about divorce. You are choosing the person you want to be with for life, with whom you want to build a home and perhaps a family.

You wouldn't be human if you didn't have any doubts, but after the decision to marry is made and the machine is in motion doubts seem far more frightening. Most people find it hard to examine their fears to see if they are valid.

The closer it gets to the wedding day, the more money that has been spent, the more organising that has been done, the more wedding presents that have arrived, the harder it gets. When there is so much invested from all sides it becomes increasingly difficult to back out. These doubts are there even for couples who are not having a big wedding but a smaller one on their own or with a few friends or close family.

Nervousness is common even when you have made the right decision – any major life change will make you feel nervous. As with other big decisions you will be looking at all the future consequences. For instance, when you think of buying a house you look at the work that is needed to make it sound, how you will decorate it, plans for the garden and so on – major items that can take years to complete. In the same way, on the brink of marriage you see your lives together stretching out for years: your children, your homes, your old age – and this is daunting. Yet after you are married this long-term vision recedes and you take it, like everything else, a step at a time.

At any stage, however, it is only sensible to examine the doubts you have. It is better to admit to a mistake before you marry than afterwards. Ignoring the feelings of nervousness prevents you from finding out if you are doing the right thing. Difficulties between you are best looked at now, while you are in love and can sort them out amicably. If you can't or don't want to sort them out they can recur later and more forcefully.

One way to help you analyse if you are doing the right thing is to examine your reasons for marrying in the first place.

Reasons for marrying

Usually top of the list for marrying is that you are in love. But why have you chosen to do so now? Look at the reasons that follow and think about how good they are for your long-term prospects.

• **We want a place of our own.** Of course if you love each other and want to marry you will want a place of your own. Not being able to afford a place together is a reason that couples sometimes give for postponing the wedding. But are the reasons for wanting to leave where you are living now as strong as or stronger than the desire to set up home together? Counsellors find that a common reason for deciding to marry is to get away from where you are living now, particularly with very young couples.

If you are still living at home with your parents and you are not happy doing so – because you don't get on with your family, have little privacy, or your home life is otherwise unhappy – you might be rushing the decision to marry as a way of giving yourselves an escape route.

You must be sure that enough factors are right before deciding to marry. A desire to get out of a difficult situation can make you close your eyes to the possibility of problems once you are married.

● **Financial considerations.** It is as well to sort out your financial situation before marrying. Money problems can cause trouble between otherwise well-suited couples.

Money as the main reason for marrying does not form a firm basis for a relationship, however. Couples who would really rather live together because they are not quite sure of the strength of their feelings or their readiness to settle down sometimes marry because only then will their parents give them money for a home of their own.

Marrying because your partner has a lot of money is not a good reason either, unless you are compatible in more fundamental ways. The relief or excitement that having plenty of money brings wears off very soon, only to highlight the real nature of the relationship.

Similarly, some women are keen to marry so that they can give up work and be supported. This can work fine if it is what you both want, but it should be discussed first. It does not make for happiness if it is the main reason.

● **He or she proposed.** The decision to marry often evolves during a relationship and the proposal can be a formality, or there may never

---

❗——————— *Task* ———————

Marriage will . . .

Think of how you would like things to be after you marry, and make yourself three lists under these headings:

Marriage will make me . . .

Marriage will make you . . .

Marriage will make us . . .

Look at each other's lists and talk about the points you have both raised.

❗

even be one. But occasionally one of you proposes out of the blue before the issue of marriage has arisen naturally. There is nothing wrong with this so long as the acceptance and the decision to marry are given careful thought by both of you.

For some people the fact that anyone wants to marry them is enough. If you are unsure of yourself and have worried that no one will ever want to marry you it is possible to be carried along by the strength of your partner's feelings. This can happen at any age, but the fear of being left on the shelf can increase with age. For some people the idea of loneliness is so frightening that anyone is better than no one at all.

Gratitude is not the best basis for a relationship. Like excitement over money it does wear off, and can be replaced by resentment. To have a happy life together after marriage means that there must be solid good feelings between you.

When the pursuer is madly in love with you and is determined to marry you it can be an intoxicating time. You are likely to feel much more than gratitude – the excitement of being loved can feel very similar to being in love yourself. But there is a shift once the relationship settles down. The joy of capture can last for some time, with the pursuer thrilled at finally having 'got' you – but, again, this does wear off, which is when the intense loving courting goes too. This is fine and normal – but if your decision to marry is based on this state continuing you will be disappointed.

● **We want to have children.** This is one of the most common reasons for marrying, particularly with couples who have been living together. It is a very good reason if you have already proved the strength of your feelings and commitment to one another. Having children is a serious step and your children deserve that you have the best possible relationship between you.

Having children to cement a rocky relationship is not a good idea. Problems between you will not be resolved in this way, and sometimes they get worse.

❛――――――――Talking point ――――――――

Children

Discuss your attitudes to having children. Do you want any? How many do you want? When should you have your first? Do you have a preference for boys or girls – and if so why?

❜

Marrying because the woman has become pregnant accidentally also happens quite often. This can work out fine if your relationship is good in other ways, but can cause real problems if it is not. An accidental pregnancy puts pressure on good relationships and can cause real rifts in relationships that are not solid. This is not the place to go into the alternatives of single motherhood, abortion or adoption, but within the limits of your beliefs, these alternatives should be looked at too.

Occasionally one of you wants marriage because you want children although you have not discussed this with your partner. Often this is because you assume you both feel the same way. Your views on children should be discussed before you marry. These views can and do change with time, but you would be wise to know how each other feels now.

● **Marriage will improve our relationship.** Couples who are not getting on well together sometimes hope that making it legal will help. This is often the case if one of you wants to marry more than the other and it is causing friction between you. But while one of you might feel more secure after the wedding the other might equally feel more trapped – causing a different set of problems.

This also happens when one of you feels the other slipping away. Offering marriage at this time can help temporarily, but the reasons that caused you to draw apart are likely to remain. You must be sure in your own minds that the problems you are experiencing as a couple before marriage can be sorted out between you, and not expect the wedding alone to make them go away.

● **Sex outside marriage is wrong.** This is a less common reason for marriage than it used to be, nevertheless it is still important to some people for religious, cultural or other reasons. Again it is important to find out how well suited you are in other ways before you take the step of marrying. Strong sexual attraction that you are not allowed to satisfy can make you feel even more madly in love and make it hard to think straight about your relationship.

● **What other people think.** Pressure from parents and other people whose opinions you care about can be a strong factor in your decision to marry. Mild, but constant, pressure can be brought to bear on you when you are living together by people asking when you are going to make it official or implying that you don't love each other enough. Practical factors sometimes count too – one of you might be in a job where they prefer their employees to be married.

Doubts before a wedding can be magnified if you have any sense that you are being pushed into it by other people's expectations rather than by your own desire.

!————————— *Task* —————————

I like it

Think about your relationship *now* before you are married. What do you like best about it and what does your partner do that gives you most pleasure? This can be anything from buying you presents, calling you by a funny name or even something sexual. Make two lists

I like it when we . . .
I like it when you . . .

Look through your lists and tick anything you hope will continue after you are married. Put a cross by anything you think will have to stop. Look at each other's lists and do the same thing – tick what you think will continue, cross what you don't want or expect to do any more.

!

• **Arranged marriages.** In certain communities of our multi-cultural society arranged marriages still happen. These can be very successful when both of you believe this is the right way for marriages to be decided. Compatibility is likely to be excellent when you come from a community where your expectations of your future life together and the roles you must play match exactly. A marriage that is sensitively arranged by people who know you both well is sometimes less haphazard than waiting to fall in love, which, as we have seen, doesn't always lead you to the right partner. People in successful arranged marriages don't miss out on falling in love – they report that this often follows marriage and can be as blissful as anyone else's experiences.

Problems arise when one or both of you have absorbed the expectations of the mainstream of the society in which you live. Then you might wish to choose your own partner, or indeed you might have fallen in love with someone whom your community would not allow you to marry. This problem is outside the scope of this book – but you could benefit from counselling, which will help you sort out mixed feelings.

• **It is about time.** This reason is not necessarily as weak as it sounds. If you have tested your relationship to your own satisfaction, marriage can be a practical and logical next step.

It needs looking at more carefully, however, if it arises from some outside pressure, for instance all your friends are getting married and you don't want to be left behind. Women especially often receive the unspoken message that there is something wrong with them if they are not married by a certain age. This can result in agreeing to marry the best man around at the moment, whatever the state of your relationship. He might very well be the best man for you – but you must be sure.

● **We want to be together.** Another good reason for marrying if you have discovered that you are compatible and have a good relationship that has lasted beyond feeling in love.

But as with the other reasons you must think around why you feel like this now. If you are not quite sure about the strength of your relationship but choose to marry (rather than, say, live together) because of your parents or your religious beliefs, these pressures might be hurrying you into a hasty decision.

The best reasons were all explored in the last chapter: compatibility, similarity of expectations and the ability to communicate with each other on all levels, physically, emotionally and verbally – or at least the willingness to develop the capacity to do so.

Your doubts

If, after thinking about your reasons, real doubts are raised in your mind it does not mean you should not marry. What it does mean is that you should talk about your doubts together and see what needs tackling. It also means that you should think further about your compatibility and how you communicate. Reading the chapter on Communication and doing the tasks and quizzes can help at this time and will allow you to clarify the state of your relationship. Going to see a Relate counsellor if you need extra help over problems is also a sensible step – there is a limit to what you can do by yourself. Premarital counselling is not wasted and can give you the tools to cope with problems in your relationship for years after the wedding.

One counsellor saw a couple before they married – still a relatively rare thing for couples to do. Ellen and Peter came to see her in December saying, 'We were going to get married next May but things are going wrong between us and we don't know whether to go ahead.'

Ellen was a strong-minded, quick-tempered, outgoing girl who had developed these qualities in order to stand up to her father, who was overbearing and restrictive. Peter was shy and dreamy. He came from a large family where, because he was quiet, he had been rather ignored and pushed out by his more difficult brothers and sisters. They had fallen in love with their opposite personalities. Peter was the kind and gentle man that Ellen had wanted to marry – so different from her hated father.

Peter was attracted to Ellen's forcefulness and positive character and the attention she showered on him. But in the run-up to the wedding they were finding that these very characteristics were causing problems between them. Ellen had become irritated by Peter's apparent weakness and failure to support her. He was confused by her quick temper and seesaw emotions.

Because these problems were new, and the couple were still in love, the counsellor found that they were willing to look at how their personalities had grown out of their different family experiences. Both were ready to see that for the relationship to become better balanced they needed to 'borrow' from each other the characteristics that had initially attracted them – indeed they saw that it could only work if Peter learned to be more assertive and Ellen learned to be more tolerant and patient. They came for six sessions of counselling, which included the counsellor giving them tasks to practise new ways of behaving together. By the end of this time, because the goodwill, love and commitment were there, the relationship had improved immensely. At the end of counselling they reset the wedding day.

It's not too late to change your mind

But if at the end of your soul-searching serious doubts are still there, you must have the courage to call the wedding off or postpone it. The money spent, the disappointment of family and friends, or the misery of your partner are, finally, less important than going into a marriage half-heartedly or with deep misgivings. Building a good and happy relationship needs effort and commitment from both of you and if it is not there you are storing up problems for yourselves.

Deciding not to marry is a hard thing to do. Another counsellor also saw a couple before their marriage. The man involved was older and had recently been divorced. He was obviously still suffering from the hurts caused by his first marriage. She was young and passionately in love with him. There were many problems in their relationship, not least, as the counsellor saw at first hand, that he picked on her to the point of cruelty, even during the counselling sessions. When the counsellor gently tried to draw their attention to what was happening between them, it was the woman who refused to pay attention to what this might mean for their future together. After two sessions of counselling they dropped out, still planning to marry, and still carrying their problems with them. As the counsellor observed, breaking up is hard, but ultimately less hard than suffering an unhappy marriage.

6 ================Talking point ================

Your vows

Do you know what your marriage vows are going to be? Discuss them together and what they mean to you. If you don't know what they will be, make up your own, discussing your suggestions with each other.

THE WEDDING DAY

As we have discussed, the run-up to the wedding can be a stressful time, but if all goes well it should be a lovely day. Many brides, particularly, aim to make this 'the happiest day of my life'. Sometimes, however, the excitement, the exhaustion from the preparation, nerves, shyness, worry over doubts and other strains mean that you don't get all the pleasure you had hoped for from either the ceremony or the celebrations afterwards.

The important point to remember is that if things do go wrong or the day is less successful than you expected there will be other happy days to follow. What counts is what you do within the marriage not the wedding day itself.

It is on the day itself that families and friends can make themselves felt in different ways. If strong-minded relatives and close family ties are involved they will be obvious at the wedding. Troubles with family and friends during the wedding can be symbolic of troubles that will need handling later – they are highlighted at the wedding not caused by it. For instance if the bride's mother is snobbish or the groom's father is mean, or the best man (his best mate) has a tendency to get drunk, all these elements can show up.

THE HONEYMOON

Much store is set by the honeymoon. It is something you both look forward to, even if you haven't been equally keen on the idea of the wedding day itself. At the very least you expect to have a great holiday at the beginning of your life together – something to symbolise the rightness of your love and your decision to marry.

Some honeymoons are as good as you imagine, but if yours is not it can be a bitter disappointment. A less than perfect honeymoon – or one that at times is downright bad – can make you wonder at the wisdom of your decision. It is worth looking at why things might not go well.

Remember what you have just been through. Even a modest wedding is stressful. After a period of stress you tend to collapse: you need a rest. What you are usually expecting is a highly sexual, very romantic time, but often one or both of you just hasn't got the energy.

There are other points that can add to your unease. It may be the first time you've been alone together without any friends around. You are thrown into each other's company for twenty-four hours a day – not a relaxing prospect if, up to now, you have never spent more than a few hours at a time together. At the back of your mind can be the fear that you will now find out that you bore each other or don't get on. The new wife might never have let her man see her without make-up before and wonder if he will still find her attractive. Any doubts that you repressed once the wedding machine was set in motion can now start to surface. With the wedding over you can't keep them pushed down forever.

Sex might be different from what you expected too. Even couples who have been sleeping together can find that their sex life changes after the wedding, even as early on as the honeymoon. If you have not lived together, time in each other's company will have been precious. You will have given each other your full, loving concentration – which will have helped to put you both in the mood for sex. Now with all the time in the world the urgency goes, and with it some of the wooing. The woman can find it more difficult to feel ready for sex. Without the stimulation and excitement of snatched moments sex can seem more ordinary.

The extra edge of excitement can also go for some when marriage removes the 'illicit' feeling of unmarried sex. Some couples need the stimulation of doing something they feel is 'not quite right'. Even couples who have been living together can notice this happening. These matters will be dealt with fully in the chapter on Sex.

The point of mentioning these problems is to show that they are not unique to you and that if they happen you should not assume that you have made a mistake in marrying. Difficulties that arise, sexual or otherwise, are part of settling down together, and helping you to recognise and deal with them effectively is the aim of this book.

THE FIRST YEAR OF MARRIAGE

In this brief look at your first year of married life, we are again going to concentrate on potential difficulties, although they are by no means the experience of every newly married couple. We are also going to ignore the couples who have their first child within this year, as the experience of having your first child and its impact on your marriage is looked at in detail later on.

Setting up home together when you are very much in love and have no real responsibilities except to your relationship can be a glorious time, and many couples look back on their early married life with great pleasure. But learning to live together in a way that suits you both calls for some adjustments, and can seem an anticlimax after the wedding and honeymoon, so it is not surprising that other couples can go through some bumpy times.

These are the main factors that can make the first year difficult.

● **Leaving your family.** Some young couples marry straight from home, without ever having lived alone or with anyone other than members of their family. Moving in with just one other person, however much in love you are, is a big change. The change from being looked after in the family environment you know so well to living with one other person and sharing in a new way takes some getting used to. It can be frightening, particularly if, at the back of it all, is the feeling that 'I've done it now!' and there is no immediate possibility of changing your mind.

● **Moving.** Moving into any new place is recognised as being a major cause of stress. On the list of the most common stress-causing factors, moving is very near the top. It involves thought all the time, even over such mundane things as where the light switches are or which direction the lavatory is when you get up in the middle of the night. On top of that there is the effort of putting your home straight and making it as you want it. Add to this the fact that getting married is, in itself, also stressful, as is learning to live together, and it is easy to see that you are sometimes going to feel tired and anxious.

● **Getting to know each other.** The majority of couples really get to know each other after they marry. Even those who have lived together have a lot more to find out as they move into a situation that means settling down and planning for the future. It would be a miracle if everything you found out about your partner struck you as perfect.

Practical matters around the home are also involved: how you divide the work, and your basic pattern of living, how good you are in the morning, for instance. Two individuals settling down together are bound to have differences that needs sorting out.

● **Money.** Money is likely to be short to begin with, and there's even less of it if you are buying somewhere to live. Young couples who have lived at home and have had jobs often find that the money they turned over to their parents was not representative of the true costs and that they have much less now.

Money worries, and distress over not being able to buy what you want or need are made far worse if you find out that you have different attitudes to money. You need to come to some agreement on credit, saving, extravagance and financial priorities, or it will continue to be a source of conflict even when money is in plentiful supply.

● **Falling out of love.** The first year of marriage often coincides with the time that you will naturally be moving out of the 'in love' stage and developing a different kind of love. If you haven't been expecting this it can be disturbing to do so once you are married; it can raise fresh doubts about the wisdom of your decision to marry. Because it comes as a shock you might find your feelings difficult to discuss and see problems as issues that must be avoided rather than tackled. Understanding that this is normal can help you cope with these emotions and the problems that arise, particularly by helping you to recognise the need to work on the way you communicate with each other.

● **Your doubts.** Doubts that did not surface during the wedding or honeymoon can plague you now. Those you had before won't go away on their own. Some people feel temporarily trapped and others a passing wistfulness about the fact that their options are no longer open, that they can't look at members of the opposite sex in the same way.

Doubts large and small are still normal at this time but you can use the impetus of your commitment to work through any that are caused by real differences.

● **Expectations.** Most of the problems that arise during this year are caused firstly by your own unconscious expectations of what marriage will do for you, and secondly by the differing expectations of your partner.

When you marry somebody you love you expect to be the happiest you have ever been. You expect the immediate aftermath to be a magic time. You certainly think that the wedding and setting up home together will be good, and, if you are young, you will feel that becoming independent from your parents will add to your happiness. If all this does not make you entirely happy you can feel guilty and worried. Knowing that a lot of money has been spent to 'send you off' or help you set up home also makes you feel that happiness is your duty as well as your right.

If things don't work out as you expect an added difficulty is feeling that you can't talk about it. How do you admit to family and friends that you are not happy? This is often something you can't share with your partner either – especially if your feelings are connected to problems between you. All this can make it a very lonely time for you.

'I thought it would all be different after the wedding,' is something counsellors occasionally hear. This is said by people who might have had doubts or difficulties before but thought that the wedding was going to put everything right. What a wedding does is marry you to your partner – no more and no less, and if you expect anything else there is bound to be disappointment.

Different expectations of the married state, as discussed in the previous chapter, will usually surface during the first year. An example of this is Jenny and Phil, who had a lot of getting to know each other to do.

They married when she was twenty-one and he was twenty-three. They had had a marvellous relationship when they were going out with each other. Jenny was a bright, vivacious girl who was something of a star in their group. She had not wanted to live with Phil before they married, though they had a sexual relationship, which both of them said was very good.

They found a flat before they married and Phil moved in six months before the wedding to get it ready. After the wedding, when Jenny moved in, there was immediate friction between them. He had developed a rather quiet routine and suddenly there was Jenny being her bubbly, noisy self around the place. She was a girl who needed to talk a great deal about what she was thinking and feeling and about everything that happened to her. Previously her mother had been the listener and now she expected Phil to take her mother's place. Phil, who had enjoyed Jenny's chattering in small doses felt swamped.

All this resulted in Phil withdrawing and becoming rather cool in the relationship. This was made worse by the fact that he considered that as he had now 'got' Jenny he no longer needed to treat her as someone special. As he reasoned to the counsellor they eventually went to see, 'Now we're together all the time, why bother to go out?

Jenny wanted to be taken out and to continue their pleasant social life. She liked to go out with their friends, to have a reason for dressing up and looking nice. She felt that since their marriage the relationship had become drab and miserable. With the romance gone Jenny went off sex; Phil, on the other hand, assumed she should be ready for sex whenever he was – they were married weren't they? He didn't feel that he should need to court her or put her in the mood for making love.

Dealing with problems

Jenny and Phil felt that if the first year was bad then it could only get worse. Instead they were helped to see that it was a year of adjustment and that they couldn't live out their separate views of marriage without taking each other into account.

It is important for any couple with similar problems to see that a difficult first year gives you the potential to make matters between you very much better. It is essential not to ignore a problem whenever it surfaces. Angry feelings can start now which will simmer for years if they are not looked at and dealt with. Ultimately the better the communication between you the less problems are able to harm your relationship – and that is the subject of the next chapter.

?——————————Quiz——————————

Money

How similar is your attitude to money? Do this quiz to see if your answers coincide.

Your earnings
Which comes closest to the way you handle your earnings?
a) You know your outgoings and you budget, using what is left over for treats; b) Much of your earnings go to pay off debts incurred since the last pay packet; c) You pay bills on time, but don't know what you usually spend and don't budget; d) You always save something – you would rather give up treats to do this.

A windfall
If you suddenly won £10,000 what are you most likely to do with it?
a) Put it all on deposit; b) Buy some shares; c) Use it all for something wildly extravagant or presents for loved ones; d) Save most and have fun with the rest; e) Put it as a deposit on a house

Money is . . .
Pick three that you agree with
a) for security and using sensibly; b) for enabling you to do as you want; c) the root of all evil – people are too materialistic; d) essential – you can't have too much; e) all right in its place – better to be 'comfortable' than rich; f) only a problem if you have too little; g) the way to gain respect – people only take notice of you if you have it; h) for spending while you are young enough to enjoy it; i) for using for the common good.

——————————————————————————?

4

COMMUNICATION

The key to unlocking almost any relationship problem, however severe, is good, effective communication. Most couples know this. Women have read about it many times in magazine articles devoted to relationships and their difficulties. Communicate more, couples are told, and things will get better. Relate counsellors know this is far easier said than done. Most of Relate's work with troubled couples goes into showing them how to listen, how to talk, even how to argue, so that their relationships improve. It ought to be simple, but learning how to communicate effectively is surprisingly difficult. It means looking very carefully at your basic ways of behaving and sometimes breaking lifetime habits of everyday living. It requires great courage at times to examine your own thoughts and feelings and find ways to express them, and also to listen to and respect your partner's thoughts and feelings – some of which will be new or distressing to you.

Every couple coming to Relate has some trouble with communication, even though many of them are highly intelligent and articulate people. Being able to express ideas clearly is often little help when it comes to unearthing and revealing your emotions, especially when they concern delicate matters such as sex. Most of this book concentrates on heterosexual couples, and mainly those who choose to marry, as this reflects the majority of people who come to Relate for counselling. But other couples are welcome too: those who are living together, or consider themselves close even if they don't live together. Homosexual couples also come for counselling, as do single people trying to sort out what went wrong in past relationships. This chapter is for anyone in any kind of relationship, or anyone who wants to be in one. Communication difficulties are at the heart of most problems, whatever the nature of your relationship.

There are many communication tasks in this chapter and even the simple-sounding ones are difficult. If you have tried some of the tasks in the earlier chapters you will already be aware of how hard it can be to talk honestly together, even when you are talking about good feelings. The tasks that help you to delve into your past and some of your deeper, subconscious feelings can be even harder, and sometimes painful. You might find this doubly so in this chapter, particularly if you are looking at it because your relationship is in trouble. Communicating in new ways involves change and that in itself can be painful, as can realising new things about yourself and your partner.

If the tasks prove too hard to do it doesn't mean you have failed. What it can mean is that you need to talk to a trained counsellor with an organisation such as Relate. Counsellors can help you unravel uphelpful matters from the past and also ease you into new communication habits in a way that won't make things worse for you. Sometimes trying to do it on your own – particularly when your relationship is a battleground or one of you is too much in charge – can be impossible. Many couples whose counsellors are helping them to talk together in new ways only do so in their sessions until matters improve. Trying new ways of communicating on their own is too disturbing.

Looking at events from your past can also be too painful to bear without trained help. Sometimes one of you will find some aspect of your past so hurtful you won't want to face it. People say, 'I don't want to talk about the past. Let's start afresh now.' But ignoring past events that are stopping you from being happy now means that you can never put them behind you. Careful counselling allows you to approach them safely and use the memories positively.

? _____ **Quiz** _____

Feelings

Look at these lists of feelings. Imagine a man having them. Which would you not respect him for? Put an M by these. Look at them again. Which would you find disturbing in a woman? Put a W by these. Which five feelings are you aware of having most often yourself? Compare your ideas with your partner.

Angry/loud	*Sad*	*Gentle/happy*	*Insecure*
Boisterous	Sad	Soft	Uneasy
Proud	Scared	Loving	Uncomfortable
Angry	Lonely	Pleased	Flustered
Contemptuous	Trapped	Contented	Inadequate
Daring	Grieved	Kind	Hesitant
Frustrated	Weepy	Satisfied	Confused
Jealous	Miserable	Excited	Stupid
Discontented	Frightened	Glad	Awkward
Aggressive	Bored	Caring	Embarrassed
Challenging	Depressed	Receptive	Silly

?

The benefits of good communication

When you start communicating honestly and fully every aspect of your relationship can develop and improve. It is never too late for this, as one counsellor found with Elsie and Alf, a couple in their seventies.

When Elsie first came for counselling there was no relationship left to improve. She and Alf had separated and had no thoughts of getting back together. Elsie had only come to Relate because her nerves were bad and her doctor had referred her to the local centre to see if they could help her come to terms with the end of her forty-five-year marriage.

The marriage had been fraught with difficulties. Sex had never been good, but they had had two children. Their daughter had died eight years earlier of breast cancer. For the past few years Alf had become increasingly violent until, in the end, Elsie had made him leave. She was still living in their house but he had found a small flat.

After the first two sessions with Elsie alone, the counsellor asked if Alf would be prepared to join them so that a complete picture of the relationship could emerge. Alf agreed, and then continued to come with Elsie. It was a relief to both Elsie and Alf to have someone to talk to about their problems.

Weeks of talking with the counsellor seemed to bring them no nearer to understanding their life together and where things had gone wrong, so one week the counsellor asked them to do a task she called the 'line of life'. They were each to take a sheet of paper and draw a line across the middle. Above the line, in chronological order, they were to write the good things they could remember from the past ten years, and below the line their bad or unhappy memories. When they returned the next week Alf reported that he had been unable to do this task: he found it hard to think about feelings or separate them into good or bad. Elsie, on the other hand, had done it – but she had not stopped with the last ten years. She had represented her whole life from the time she was born on several sheets of paper. Alf agreed to share Elsie's line of life and make his own comments.

For Elsie unhappy feelings were part of her earliest memories, but she had never talked about them. Now it emerged that her brother had sexually interfered with her from the time she was a baby. He had crept into her room after she was in bed and had touched her in ways she hated and knew were wrong. Elsie had never told Alf this. When Alf entered the picture on the line of life the below-the-line unhappy feelings were all to do with sex.

What had sex made her feel? asked the counsellor. Uncomfortable, frightened and out of control Elsie remembered. For Alf this was an astounding revelation. 'Is that why you always had to have the light on and I had to go straight into intercourse without touching you anywhere?'

he asked. Elsie agreed that was so. The dark and any kind of intimate touching had reminded Elsie of the horrible episodes with her brother. For all those years Alf had felt a failure and sex between them had been quick and unsatisfactory, but the reasons had nothing to do with them – they were all rooted in the past. They were hard for Elsie to remember or admit to and it took great courage for her to do so.

As they progressed through Elsie's line of life they came to the point, eight years ago, when their daughter had died. This had been terrible for both of them, but Alf had 'taken it like a man'. Now, after Elsie's admissions about her past – and Alf's own churned-up feelings surrounding their separation – he could not keep a 'stiff upper lip' any more. He went to pieces in the counselling room, weeping and doubling-up in agony at the memory. It was these held in feelings that had stopped him from being able to look at or remember any other feelings – and had caused him to become violent towards Elsie.

After this session they decided to try again together. Alf moved back in and everything changed. Within the counselling sessions they continued to work at finding ways to tell each other about their feelings and trying to understand each other's point of view. For the first time sex between them started to become good. The counsellor said, 'I knew their ages but it was as if they were in their forties. They were at the beginning of a new relationship. There was more acceptance, more love, more space – and, because of that, more togetherness. The change was the most dramatic I have seen.'

Not all changes in communication will have such sudden and dramatic results – but if both of you are willing the benefits can be just as good. Couples who have found new ways to relate to each other find that these lessons have effects on other areas of their lives too. Some habits of good communication seem like a 'trick' or rather false in the beginning, but after a while they become part of your way of acting and feel quite normal. Couples often report how these 'tricks' work in other situations: with their children, with their parents, at the office and among friends. The tricks are almost all to do with working out what you really feel and want and explaining it in such a way as to make the other person understand. They involve encouraging other people to do the same, and respecting their different feelings and needs. Finally they involve coming to agreements with which you can both live. They are tricks that make all your relationships run more smoothly, not just those with your closest family.

❛————————Talking point ————————

In a nutshell

The essence of good communication is contained in these three points:

1. Telling exactly how you feel
2. Listening to what the other says
3. Accepting your partner's opinions and feelings even when they are different from your own

   Discuss why you think these elements make for good communication.

❜

SEPARATE WORLDS

What does effective communication actually do? It is the only way you can show anyone who you are, what you want and why you behave as you do. It is the only way you can really understand what makes someone else tick. Without these elements problems can crop up between you and it is difficult to understand why they have happened (or why they have happened *now*) and, because of this, however much you try it is hard to solve them.

This is because we are all very complicated. Everything we do, say and think now is tied up with the experiences of our entire lives. Two people can have an apparently identical experience but both will view it differently because of the different feelings that they bring to it. For instance, imagine a couple taking a walk by the sea on a fine summer's day. It makes one of them feel happy and light-hearted, touching off old memories of fun at the seaside as a child. The other, however, never learnt to swim well and finds the sea threatening and hostile and it brings up old feelings of being inadequate and frightened.

This might seem an extreme example, but to an extent this happens at all levels in your life. Only you will feel and think exactly your emotions and thoughts. Even at moments of great togetherness with your loved one – making love, for example, both of you can feel happy and loving but it will be in slightly different ways, connected as it is to many other feelings and memories conscious or forgotten.

Because you are an individual, different from anyone else alive, no one can ever know what it is like to be you. Each of us inhabits our own separate world, most of it hidden from view. People know what you look like, hear what you say and watch what you do. They can draw some conclusions from this, some of them true. They can fall in love with what they think you to be. But only you can show them the whole picture. The only way someone can enter your world and understand what you are like is by means of you talking to them and showing them. The only way you can truly know someone else is by listening to their own explanations of their feelings and thoughts. True love is about making the effort to understand the different world a loved one inhabits and to respect the individuality within it. True love is trusting someone else enough to show yourself entire, without protecting yourself by keeping parts hidden. A truly loving relationship is one in which you both make efforts to understand the other's world and allow each other to be different and separate.

Knowing the 'secret you' is hard enough for you to do, as we saw in Chapter 2. Explaining it to someone else is even harder. It is never entirely possible to understand how life looks and feels to someone else however carefully they explain it, so listening and making the effort to understand is the hardest of all. These are some of the reasons why communicating is so difficult.

Men should . . . women should . . .

Another reason people find it so difficult to show even their closest partners what they are thinking and feeling is that most of us are brought up to believe that certain ways of behaving are right and some emotions and thoughts are wrong.

Exactly which emotions are wrong are considered different for men and women. Men grow up thinking that it is all right for them to be strong and occasionally aggressive but that there is something wrong about feeling frightened, weak, weepy, vulnerable or sentimental. Women are brought up to believe that it is all right to show all the softer range of emotions but that anger and any of the more pushy and aggressive emotions are wrong. Years of training, conscious or not, produces grown men and women who are best at recognising or expressing such emotions and thoughts as are considered acceptable and who find it hard to acknowledge even to themselves that other feelings are there too.

But every one of us feels every one of the entire range of emotions, and must do so to be a fully rounded, effective and *adult* human being. Everyone feels anger from time to time and everyone feels fear. Your personality type dictates how strongly you feel the variety of emotions: there will be some you experience particularly powerfully and others that you will be better able to handle, but they will all be triggered off inside you at some time.

If you think that it is wrong to feel certain emotions you are likely to bury them so deeply that you are no longer even aware of them, or you might unconsciously change them into something else. A man who believes he should never feel weakness or fear can quickly change these emotions into anger. A woman who is scared of feeling angry can weep or feel depressed instead.

This also happens if you find an emotion too hard to bear. You will have your own way of changing a difficult emotion into one that you feel you should have and can handle – and the better you are at doing this the harder it is for you to find out what it is you are really feeling.

If you think this is nonsense then you are not alone. Haven't we just said that you are the only person who can really know what you are feeling? How dare someone tell you that you are feeling something quite different from what you know to be the truth! But it is not nonsense. Time and again in counselling people who are very sure they know themselves and their own feelings uncover the fact that underneath the surface are emotions that they didn't even know they had. This is always painful. You don't know that you have them for the very good reason that you find them difficult to handle or even frightening. The better the job you have done in keeping them down the more frightening they are. If you have never let them out, you have no idea what might happen if you did: perhaps you would lose control, go mad or spend your whole time crying about some unbearable sadness you have just re-discovered.

Luckily this is not what happens. Once you have refound a frightening, powerful emotion and experienced the painful difficulty of knowing that this is how you really feel, it starts to lose its strength. Buried feelings, like weeds with only their leaves cut off, remain strong under the surface. It is only by pulling them out, roots and all, that you tackle the problem. It is only when you deal with weeds effectively that your garden can grow to its full glory – weeds stifle the growth of better plants. It is only when you find and tackle your hidden emotions that you can feel all the range of pleasant emotions too. Keeping a feeling buried takes a lot of unconscious energy which leaves less left over for feelings of happiness.

Unlike weeds though, you don't kill off a buried emotion when you discover it is there. It loses its power but it doesn't go away. What does happen is that it becomes controllable. Once you have unearthed the powerful, unbearable anger, for instance, which you have hidden away it becomes smaller and more bearable. Now you can feel appropriate anger at the right moments and *you* can control it – it doesn't take you over.

Knowing that this is so doesn't make it any easier, unfortunately. Most people prefer to carry on the way they are. They have found a way of operating that works perfectly well for them, so why rake up old miseries? Other people continue to believe that these ideas about buried and forgotten emotions are nonsense. The pity is that half of good communication involves knowing yourself well and explaining yourself to others – without it effective communication can't happen.

You cry for me and I'll shout for you

It is quite common for two people, both burying different emotions, to fall in love. Sometimes part of the unconscious attraction is that one of them is feeling and expressing the very emotions that the other has hidden away and forgotten.

This can result in a relationship that works, sometimes for years; the 'marital fit' that we talked about in Chapter 2. A man who won't allow himself to feel fear or panic might be very drawn to a woman who becomes weepy and out of control when things go wrong. When he feels a flicker of fear he says or does something that makes his wife react by becoming hysterical. When this happens he somehow feels better – he feels strong and in control, and perhaps even angry or irritated by his wife's behaviour. Neither of them has the slightest idea what they are doing. This same woman might tell herself and others that she never gets angry – her husband is the one who is always losing his temper. When something inside her starts to feel a little angry she finds herself doing or saying something that provokes an angry outburst from her husband. This makes her cry – and perhaps she hates him for it – but her angry feelings have gone away and she is dealing with something she understands: sadness.

This is quite a striking division of emotions, but counsellors find that many couples 'fit' together in such obvious or less obvious ways. Sometimes it works out very happily for them – but not necessarily for ever. The fit continues to work as long as both of you continue to divide emotions into 'his' and 'hers', but if one of you changes in any way it can make the other feel seriously disturbed, and then the problem flares. The one who has changed might now need a different sort of 'fit' or perhaps have reached a better understanding of his or her emotions and be beginning to acknowledge and accept some of the hidden feelings – but the other doesn't like the change or can't or won't see that the same is also true for him or her.

Because you need the other person to behave in ways that suit you – to think and feel what fits in with you – the fit does not allow individuality or development and without these a relationship will slowly die or be broken up by a crisis.

A counsellor talked about the case of Fiona and George, to whom this happened. Fiona had agoraphobia and could not leave the house without George. Many other matters would also trigger off an anxiety condition that would leave her shaking and sometimes bedridden. George was marvellous. He was absolutely supportive. He even lost one job because he left to be by Fiona's side in the middle of the day once too often. He cossetted her. He drove her everywhere. He said he would do anything to help her become better. Through counselling Fiona did start to improve. But as she did so, George started to become resentful and anxious. The counsellor tried to help him to get in touch with the side of himself that needed Fiona to be sick: he needed the belief that he was strong and protective, but he couldn't sustain it unless she was weak. As she became stronger the weakness in himself that he was denying began to show. They stopped their sessions at this stage because George was convinced that the counselling was responsible for the marriage becoming shaky.

The 'fit' between couples can work for many years until some change forces a crisis. At this point couples may know that something is wrong but not know what to do about it. The way through this is by developing communication skills and by changing habits of behaviour. Some of the tasks that follow can help, but as we have said before, if they are too difficult to tackle alone counselling could be the answer. If both of you acknowledge a need to change and are willing to work on yourselves as well as on your relationship, radical improvement can follow.

STARTING WELL

Before we look at the problems, however, there will be some of you who are reading this before you have trouble between you, and who want to set up now a pattern of communicating that is helpful.

This is a responsible attitude which will stand you in good stead. No one ever teaches you about relationships. You learn to speak, but not to talk – not in the way we have been examining here. No one bothers about how you listen – beyond checking that your hearing is healthy. Neither skill occurs naturally and both need developing. Everything you know about relationships comes from what you observed while you were growing up, and unless the people around you were very skilled you have probably not learnt the most helpful patterns of behaviour. More than that, what you did learn were patterns that worked in your own family but which will not necessarily work in another situation. When you start living with someone else you have not been trained to make the best of it.

When you are in love you want to talk to each other and you want to listen; you usually like to talk about everything under the sun. This is a good start and something you should hang on to as your relationship changes and develops with the passing years. Valuing your partner's opinions is part of valuing the kind of person he or she is, which is an element of good communication.

Arguing also comes into this. You are not going to think alike on every subject and learning how to disagree without a battle of wills is a skill. Having arguments about matters which are not greatly important to you allows you to try out various means of handling disagreements. Then when an issue comes up that you really feel deeply about you will be better able to handle it in positive rather than destructive ways. All this is dealt with later in the chapter.

❛━━━━━━━━━ Talking point ━━━━━━━━━

Your relationship bank account

It is useful to think about your relationship as a bank account, into which you pay in and take out. When things are going well for you and you are acting towards each other in ways that are loving, you are making 'deposits' that keep the account healthy. When matters are going wrong or you are rowing a lot you are drawing on the good feelings that are there. When the account is empty you start to be in real trouble.

But, as with a bank account, you can make the effort to 'pay in' when things are not easy for you. Any little loving gestures or words you use with your loved one can help to build up the account even during bad times. Making a positive effort to make time to talk, listen, have fun together, or to do something kind or generous for each other keeps something in the account to tide you over rocky patches. Discuss this with your partner – are you aware of doing this already?

❜

!━━━━━━━━━ *Task* ━━━━━━━━━

Make a date

Get your diaries – or the calendar in the kitchen – and make a date each week to spend time together. This should be at least an hour of uninterrupted time, when you are not watching the television. Regularly, make one of these dates a time to go out together, say once a month. If you have children fix up a baby-sitter or ask if they can stay with friends or a member of your family. You could also join a baby-sitting circle and 'earn' an evening out by baby-sitting for someone else.

!

Talking about everyday matters

Talking about the things that happen in your day and discussing matters that interest you (as well as those to do with the home and family) are important elements in communication. Surprisingly, counsellors often discover that couples spend only a few minutes in a day talking directly to each other, and these conversations are often about everyday household matters. It is *not* surprising, therefore, that when there is something important to talk about they are out of practice and find it even more difficult than it need be.

It is easy to slip into this habit of not talking to each other about anything other than practical matters, particularly if you are busy and have a family. Couples in trouble are often advised by counsellors to consult their diaries together and fix on a time to talk – perhaps two sessions of one hour per week. Quite often couples turn up each week for their counselling sessions having failed to make that time for one reason or another. It is hard to see how they can sort out the problems in their relationships if they can't make any time to be alone. Some have so much tension between them that even an innocent remark such as 'Have you had a good day?' leads to an icy exchange starting, 'Well I'm glad you have because mine has been awful . . .'

It might seem cold to make an appointment with your partner, but it is only sensible if your lives don't easily coincide. Many happy couples do this as a matter of course. Making time to go out together is part of this and it doesn't have to cost much money: a walk in the park, or an hour or two in the pub as a regular event.

But first we have to go back to the basics of communication – talking and listening.

TALKING, LISTENING – AND HEARING

It often becomes clear to counsellors in the first session with a new couple that much of their life together (and their problem) is built on misunderstanding. This can take three main forms: they are not expressing themselves effectively, they are not listening closely to what each other says, or they are not talking much but are making assumptions about what each other thinks or feels.

Talking

Learning to talk – which usually means finding different ways to express what you want to say – is often an early task. For many people communication – or getting your point across – means saying the same things louder and more often. It is the approach some people use with foreigners: shouting words that the foreigner doesn't understand instead of choosing different, simpler, words. Finding ways to make your partner want to listen also means ditching an unhelpful manner of talking, such as blaming.

Common habits that get in the way of helpful communication

Many communication problems result from habits of which you might not even be aware. Spotting these habits and making conscious efforts to change them can make a lot of difference. See if you recognise any of these:

● **Not saying what you really mean.** The most usual example of this is not admitting that something is bothering you when it is: telling your partner that you don't mind about something when you do, or that you are quite happy when you are not. The trouble with this is that the issue goes on bothering you, but your partner can do nothing about it; he or she either believes you that nothing is the matter or, although sensing that something is wrong, has no idea why or how it can be put right. Secretly you are usually hoping that your words will be ignored while your wishes are taken into account – but it is easy to see that this is impossible until you speak the truth. One likely outcome of not doing so is that your feelings build up over months or even years until finally you explode. Having the courage to say what you feel at the time prevents it becoming a much larger, more difficult to solve problem later.

● **Making something else the issue.** This is related to the above habit in that you are not talking about whatever it is that is really bothering you. The difference is that to relieve your feelings you start complaining about something else. For instance, one woman focused on her husband's irritating habit of leaving wet towels on the bathroom floor when the real issue was that she resented always being the one to clean the house when they were both out at work all day. Often the more difficult and emotional the real problem is the more likely you are to find something small and trivial to focus on. The trouble with this is obvious: you might sort out the trivial issue, or get into an unproductive row about it, but the main problem remains untouched. The longer it does so the more emotional you will become.

● **Not talking.** This is another way of avoiding an issue that is upsetting you. Sometimes you retreat into silence, or go out, or go to bed early rather than risk talking at all; you can't trust yourself to speak in case you go over the top. Perhaps you are hiding an important issue from your partner and so find it difficult to talk about other matters. Whatever the case, you hope that the feelings will go away or that your partner will guess what is the matter and do something about it. The feelings might go away temporarily but if they are important they will return more strongly. Your partner might guess what the problem is – or, far more likely, might not.

One example of this is Eddie and Rose who apparently had a good and happy marriage. They had a boy and a girl, now both at private schools. Early on they had agreed that they were lucky to have 'one of each' so that they wouldn't have to have any more, as educating them privately was taking most of their spare money. But over the years Rose had come to yearn for another baby. She felt unable to tell Eddie that she had changed her mind, but she couldn't stop thinking about it. Slowly, their relationship began to go wrong. Rose went off sex: subconsciously she felt Eddie was selfish in wanting sex without children. She no longer wanted to go out with Eddie and they stopped having the free and happy conversations they had previously enjoyed because Rose was unable to talk about what was most on her mind: having another baby. Eddie felt confused and rejected and fell into a short, meaningless affair with his secretary, which Rose found out about. It caused a crisis, which was why they came for counselling. Neither of them knew why things had gone so badly wrong – even Rose was unaware of the real problem since she felt that wanting another baby was 'silly' given that she had two lovely children and a good lifestyle already.

After several sessions of counselling, with communication between them improving, Rose felt able to say with much difficulty and tears that she wanted another baby. Eddie was taken aback but not shocked. He said, 'I had no idea that you wanted a baby – but, of course, if you do we will!'

Oddly enough, once Eddie had said this Rose became less sure that she did want another child. Deep down she had resented Eddie not guessing what the matter was, and as she had been unable to talk about it everything else had also gone wrong. Once it was out in the open it stopped being a problem. Now that she felt free to discuss her feelings she found out that they were more mixed than she had realised. In fact, a year later their relationship was so improved that they did decide to have another child, and they sent the counsellor a postcard telling her so.

● **Nagging.** Nagging – going on and on about something that you want changed – is a common habit of *both* men and women, although some people think it is just women who nag. When you are doing this it is possible to convince yourself that you are being positive, saying what you think when you think it. But nagging is always telling someone else what you think should be done: 'You never . . .'; 'You always . . .'; 'I hate it when you . .' and so on. Saying how something makes you feel and why is an important part of communication. Telling someone how to behave is not. If the way they are behaving upsets you then you have a right to say that it has that effect. But if you are saying it over and over again then you are not communicating effectively. It is like shouting at the foreigner. Repetition won't get you where you want to be, in fact it will have the opposite effect of making the other person 'go deaf'. Different ways of handling this are dealt with later, when we look at coping with angry feelings.

● **Holding forth.** This is when you get into the habit of talking about everything that is on your mind without noticing what effect this has on your partner. Talking is a two-way process, and part of it is being aware of the interest and participation of the other. Conversations include eye contact and comments from both. 'Are you listening?' Said sharply is not enough. Nor is 'Yes, dear' a true indication that you are being listened to. These are not the worst habits of daily life, but if you fall into these traps it makes communicating difficult when what you have to say is important and emotional.

● **Changing the subject.** This can be a trick that you use whenever the topic of conversation gets too difficult or when you are just not interested in what the other has to say. This can be very frustrating for the person who is raising an emotional subject, and demoralising if it is clearly a sign that you are bored. Closing the subject is a much more honest and positive way of doing this. Saying 'I find that hard to talk about now', or 'I can't really put my mind to that at the moment', or even 'I can't get very interested in that' is less offensive than cutting in with another subject without warning.

● **Being a know-all.** Communication becomes a one-way process if one of you takes the attitude that you always know best and are always right. The most delicate area for you to consider yourself an expert is your partner's thoughts and feelings. While you might have some good ideas about your partner's motives or deepest feelings, you can't know for sure – and neither is it up to you to explain what they are. You can ask 'Is it because . . .?' or 'Are you actually feeling . . .?' but you don't have a right to insist on the accuracy of your ideas. Only your partner can find out the truth and only your partner can show you what that is. An attitude of loving acceptance will encourage your partner to open up to you, but being a Sherlock Holmes of the emotions can have the opposite effect. 'Don't psychoanalyse me!' one woman used to shout at her husband. This invasion of her most private life – her mind and her feelings – actually stopped her wanting to look at why she thought and felt as she did.

• **Disguised criticism.** There are ways and ways of saying how you feel. Doing so in a blaming fashion is really criticism. 'You make me so sad/angry/depressed!' is making the other person responsible for what you feel. As we have seen, feelings are more complicated than that, and the other person's actions are only half the story. Criticising is never the best way to get the result you want; it puts the other person on the defensive and creates extra problems rather than the solutions you hope for.

• **The way you say it.** Manner and tone of voice are very important. Sometimes *what* you say is not the issue, but the way you say it puts your partner's back up. Talking in a lecturing or patronising way can make your partner not want to hear the message. Other tones that make people switch off are anger, coldness, irony and so on.

These are some of the habits that stop you communicating effectively at the best of times. At the worst of times, when the issues are very important and emotional, they can lead to a breakdown in communication when you most need it. New ways of communicating are looked at later in the section on 'Dealing with difficult emotions', and in some of the tasks.

Listening and hearing

While some people are aware that they have problems with expressing what they want to say, most people give little thought to how effectively they listen. A 'good listener' is someone who lets another person talk and doesn't interrupt with opinions and criticism. A good listener only occasionally gives advice and very rarely does so unasked. These people are easy to talk to because you don't feel as if you are being judged, laughed at, despised or disliked. A good listener makes you feel as if what you have to say is worth listening to – that you are respected, accepted and interesting. Some people have more of a natural talent for listening than others, but all of us can train ourselves to develop the skills of a good listener. These skills are essential in improving communication with your partner, and are also helpful in getting on with the other people in your life.

Most people find listening attentively difficult unless they are really interested in what is being said. It becomes even harder when you don't like what is being said or find it disturbing and upsetting. When you are arguing or failing to put a point across then 'listening' often only means keeping quiet while you work out what to say next; you haven't really 'heard' what the other person has said.

These are some common ways in which people fail to listen properly:

- **Switching off.** This is the tactic often used by people who complain that their partners nag. While the other person is putting a lot of energy and passion into talking they let their minds wander elsewhere.

Other people do this when their partners become very emotional. Sometimes they are not even conscious they have switched off. For instance, a man whose mother used to weep a lot when he was a child might therefore find displays of unhappy emotion distressing and switch off in panic when his wife becomes upset. Or a woman whose father flew into rages at the family and who used to retreat into a world of her own when this happened might do the same when her husband becomes angry.

- **Half-listening.** This is even more common: listening with just half your attention. Your minds is on the television or the newspaper or occupied with private thoughts of your own, but you keep just enough of it open to what is being said so that you can make the occasional sensible comment.

It doesn't matter too much if the conversation is just chitchat, but some people also do this during more important conversations. They can repeat back what has been said, but they are not listening in the sense that they are not thinking about it or trying to understand what is meant.

- **Interrupting.** Not allowing someone to finish what they are saying is the opposite of good listening. It is always a sign of wanting your own point of view to prevail and not being prepared to give consideration to the other person's opinion. Couples who are having problems can find that they have bitter rows along this pattern, both interrupting and shouting over each other, neither prepared to listen or give way. Of course this means stalemate and bad feelings which can't be resolved until the pattern is broken.

- **Mind-reading.** Mind-reading is built on assumptions. Your partner is the person you believe you know best in the world, and that often includes believing you know what he or she thinks and feels. Mind-reading makes it difficult to listen: because you think you know what your partner means you don't make a real effort to hear what is being said.

This becomes even more pronounced when your relationship is in trouble. When you are at each other's throats you need to believe that you are right and your partner is wrong. Quite often you don't want to hear what the other says, unless it is what you are expecting. That means you only listen to what is said when it proves your own theory.

Mind-reading often comes up in counselling. Couples will talk about each other to the counsellor while they are both present. One will tell the counsellor what the other thinks and feels. When the counsellor checks this out it is often revealed as assumption and different from the truth.

Another aspect of this is hearing the other's words but insisting that you know he or she 'didn't mean it'. One man who didn't want children insisted that his broody wife didn't mean it when she said she did. He chose to remember her earlier doubts and ignore what she was saying.

● **Proving your point.** This is similar to mind-reading. It involves selective listening – waiting only for the words and phrases that prove your point, ignoring anything else your partner says that does not fit. This means that you can quite literally listen without hearing.

Some people also listen selectively when they cannot bear their partners to have certain feelings or ideas. A woman who needs her husband to be strong and protective will not listen properly at the moments when he is talking about weakness or fear; instead she is listening out for the moment when his tone changes and he sounds more confident again, allowing her to forget the other conversation.

● **Blocking.** Blocking what your partner says is an effective technique for avoiding listening. The harder a subject is for your partner to talk about, the easier it is to shut him or her up by criticising, sounding

! ——————————— *Task* ———————————

I want to know who you are

Make a date to talk to your partner for one hour specifically about yourselves and your feelings. Toss a coin to see who begins. Take half an hour each to talk about how you feel and what you want in life – as if you are explaining yourself to a stranger. While each person talks, the other must be silent and listen with full attention. On the half-hour you switch roles.

During this time you must not talk about your partner or your relationship, though you can talk about your past. At the end of the hour stop the conversation and don't talk about what has been said. If you want to talk about it, make a date to do so, but not for a few days.

You might be surprised at how difficult this is – particularly to listen to your partner without interruption. You will start to feel closer if you do this regularly.

A strict rule is that you must never 'use' or twist what you have heard in these sessions during an argument. If you do so you risk losing trust and closing down communication between you.

!

shocked, correcting, laughing, changing the subject, arguing, weeping, shouting, or any other ploy you can think of rather than listening. Talking about difficult and emotional matters takes courage and needs a sympathetic listener. Without this it seems safer to give up trying.

Listening techniques

Listening is important if you are truly to understand your partner. Listening generously, attentively and uncriticially is essential if your partner is going to trust you enough to tell you his or her most intimate thoughts and feelings. If you are not used to listening quietly and fully you will find it hard at first to do so without jumping in with something of your own to say, but you will improve with practice.

Giving your whole attention to someone is hard work and quite exhausting. It is no accident that most counselling sessions of any sort last about an hour: when trying to help an individual or a couple the counsellor is listening with total concentration and to do so for longer than an hour is tiring.

Listening is most difficult when you are being told things that you don't want to hear. Most people long to cut in and be reassured that the other person doesn't really think or feel the things that are being said when they are disturbing; or want to come up with arguments to make their partners change their minds.

● **Forget about yourself.** When you truly want to listen to and hear what someone is trying to say to you then you must put your own thoughts and feelings on one side while you do so. What you should be aiming for is to get a true idea of what the other person is feeling. While listening try to understand what it must be like to have those thoughts and emotions. It is not especially useful to refer it back to yourself and what you might think or feel in such a situation.

Adding your own thoughts and ideas is not helpful in enabling you to understand what the other person is feeling. Comments might block the flow, but questions can help it on.

● **Check that you are understanding.** It can be very hard to put yourself in someone else's shoes, and sometimes the explanations might not be clear enough for you to understand. Check that you are understanding what is being said by occasionally repeating back in your own words what you have heard. The person talking will tell you if you have got the sense right or not.

People who learn this technique in counselling are pleased to find what a difference it makes to their conversations. Counsellors often practise it with couples within a session. Initially it feels artificial, but the benefits of knowing that you are being listened to and that you are really hearing what your partner has to say means that it is soon incorporated more naturally into your manner of talking together.

The technique involves one person saying something and the other responding with a summary or by putting it in a different way and asking the speaker if that was what was meant. To begin with this process is slow and even short conversations can take the whole hour of counselling. But when the couple feel there has been a breakthrough in understanding they will continue to use the technique at home and will come back and report that conversations are getting better. It helps the listener more than any other technique to understand what is being said. One counsellor told of a session with a couple who were having sexual problems that began because the husband never kissed his wife during sex and this made her feel used. Had she told her husband this? the counsellor wanted to know. Many times, she said. Because it was not important to him, he chose not to listen to her words. 'What is she saying?' the counsellor asked. 'She is saying that she likes to be kissed when we make love,' he replied. 'Why do you need this?' the counsellor asked the wife. 'Because kissing makes me feel that he really loves me and then I feel tender and sexy', she replied. 'Why does she need this?' the counsellor asked the husband, and he repeated her words. Although the husband found this conversation awkward and stilted, repeating his wife's words made him think for the first time about what she was saying, and he was able to do as she wanted.

Some people can find this very hard because they add their own interpretation to the other person's words. One counsellor described a session in which a wife was trying to explain to her husband how she felt about something. He could not get it into his head, so the counsellor asked him to repeat it back to her in his own words. Twice he repeated what he believed rather than what he had heard. His wife had to say the same thing three times before he was able to repeat the true sense of what she had said. He had a strong opinion that women were illogical (like his mother) so when his wife was calm and logical he heard what he believed she 'truly meant' – something overemotional and illogical.

● **Ask for clarification.** If you are not sure that you understand tell the other person and ask if it can be put in a different way or if you can be given an example. In the same way, if your attention wanders for a moment and you realise you missed something, ask the other person to repeat it.

● **Wait to give an opinion.** Your opinions on factual matters can be relevant, but opinions on someone else's feelings and emotions are best kept to yourself. Feelings can't be changed by someone else's opinion that they are silly, immature, over-the-top, unkind, not 'real', or by any other judgement. Behaviour and actions can be controlled and changed by an effort of will but feelings come and go of their own accord. The role of a good listener is to respect absolutely the other person's right to have his or her own feelings, however 'wrong', frightening or strong they seem.

If your opinion has been asked for, resist the temptation to give it until the other person has said everything he or she wants to say. Even then, confine yourself to giving your opinion on actions and practical matters. Making someone ashamed of what he or she is feeling won't make that feeling go away – it will only make it harder for him or her to express other thoughts or feelings to you.

Understanding

The result of effective communication – talking honestly and listening attentively – is increased understanding between you. With understanding comes the recognition that your partner is not 'part of you' but a separate individual with some similarities and many differences.

Understanding is one of the main elements of a good relationship. When communicating like this becomes a part of your life together you become equipped to deal with any problems that arise. As you change – which you both will do – you are able to understand how and why the other is changing because you can talk about it and listen carefully. That means that difficulties can be negotiated and dealt with, using respect and acceptance, over a period of time.

SHOWING

Talking together is one of the main elements of good communication, but you demonstrate your love in other ways, too. One counsellor's definition of a good marriage is 'one in which you cherish each other' – and cherishing suggests physical contact as much as verbal communication.

It is important to show your partner affection physically and by acting with consideration. This is different from sex, though it is sometimes linked: women often say that they feel more sexually responsive if their husbands show them affection at other times, too: kissing, holding hands, or friendly cuddles. An example of this is Sean and Marilyn, who came for counselling because Marilyn had gone off sex. During counselling it emerged that Sean had problems with his back and had bought an orthopaedic chair. In the past they had watched television together in the evening, sitting side by side on the sofa, sometimes with

Marilyn lying with her head in Sean's lap, sometimes holding hands. Now he sat in his chair with his back to her while she sat on the sofa. This warm contact had put Marilyn in the mood for sex; now it was only Sean who ever wanted to make love.

Once they understood what had happened Sean and Marilyn decided to make the simple change of rearranging the furniture so that they could sit side by side and hold hands while they were watching television.

Sometimes you need to tell each other how you like to be shown love, and what it means to you, even when sex doesn't enter into it, as Angela and Derek found. Angela came for counselling sad and angry, saying that Derek treated her like the housekeeper. He never showed her any affection and she believed he just took her for granted. As Angela described Derek, the counsellor got the picture of a stern and unloving man. She asked if he would come for counselling too. He agreed but said that initially he would like to come on his own.

When Derek arrived, the counsellor was surprised to find him rather gentle and courteous. He explained that he was under some pressure at work and his sex drive had dwindled. What emerged was that he was frightened to get too close to Angela physically because he thought she would then want sex and he was afraid that he would be unable to perform. He was very sad about how their relationship had deteriorated. They came together for the third visit and the counsellor encouraged Derek to tell Angela what he had told her. When he had finished Angela had tears in her eyes. She said, 'All I wanted was for you to put your arm round me – I didn't want anything else!' Derek admitted that he missed the closeness too. This conversation changed Angela's feeling about Derek and the relationship.

! ══════════════ *Task* ══════════════

It makes me feel loved

Which actions or words make you feel loved and special to your partner? They can be things that your partner does, used to do, or you would like your partner to do.

Make a list of these. Men often find this harder to do than women. Give your lists to each other and discuss which you will find easy and which difficult. Keep each other's lists and try to find occasions to do what your partner would like.

!

! ════════════════════ *Task* ════════════════════

Do it for me

Make a pact where every day you take it in turns to ask your partner to do something for you that you would like. It must not be something that your partner would find unpleasant or uncomfortable. It can be very simple: allow you to choose the evening viewing on television, do the washing up, give you half an hour of peace when you come in from work, or bring you a drink in bed. It can also be something to do together: go swimming or for a walk, or weed the garden. It could be very personal, such as giving you a massage, washing your hair for you or something sexual that perhaps you used to do but haven't for a while.

Don't be surprised if you find it difficult to think of what you would like. Counsellors find many couples have lost the habit of doing things together or for each other and often have to think long and hard before they can come up with even one thing they would like.

!

! ════════════════════ *Task* ════════════════════

I've been thinking about you

One counsellor regularly gives couple the task of giving each other presents that don't cost anything yet which show love and thought. She describes how one man gave his wife an acorn, which, he explained, symbolised the walks they used to take together and enjoy and was also an object that from small beginnings grows into something big and enduring. The woman gave her husband a safety pin, saying that it was simple and serviceable yet able to unite two different things – which their efforts to mend the relationship were also doing.

Give your partner something like this – the value of it being that you have thought of each other and your relationship.

Other ideas are: a cutting from a newspaper that might interest or amuse your partner or a note in which you tell your partner something that you like or love about him or her. Aim to do this once in a while.

!

Daily habits

Simple habits that become part of daily life can make a great difference to how you get on together. Counsellors have found that apparently minor tasks – couples paying a little loving attention to each other before they part in the morning, kissing and saying goodbye in a friendly manner – have a beneficial impact on the relationship.

Similar evening rituals can help, such as giving each other some time and space to wind down before talking about what has happened in the day. This worked particularly well for one couple, who came for counselling because the wife, who was being driven mad by her husband's moods and aggression, was on the point of leaving him. The moment he walked into the house in the evening he would start on her, picking fault with everything that she did. Counselling had been suggested by his doctor, who was treating him for stress symptoms.

During counselling it emerged that he had a job as a time-and-motion expert. He was brought in to look at how people did their work and make suggestions as to how they could do it more effectively. This job made him unpopular with all but his superiors. No one liked being told that they had to change their way of operating, and he was often on the receiving end of bad feeling. By the time he came home in the evening he was very wound up and ready to take out the stress of the day on his wife.

As he talked, the husband was able to see that the fights he was picking with his wife had nothing to do with her or their relationship. The counsellor suggested that he found a way to dump the problems of the day before he started the evening afresh with his wife. The device that worked for the man was to write the names of the people he had had problems with at work on separate pieces of paper, then tear them up in little pieces and put them in the wastepaper basket, thinking over what had happened as he did so. When he had got the day's aggravations out of his system he was to forget about them until the next day, and then greet his wife as if he had just come in. This worked like a charm for them. The unnatural tension left the relationship and the wife decided to stay with her husband.

Practical changes in daily life can improve your relationship almost as much as understanding your own and your partner's motives. Some counsellors find that certain couples can't move forward out of a bad situation even if they have come to understand how they got themselves into it. In these cases the counsellors work purely with practical tasks to help the couples change their everyday behaviour.

This was the situation with Cheryl and Darren, a couple in their early twenties who had three children. They had got together when

Cheryl was sixteen and Darren seventeen and had married a year later. Their first child had been born before they married. From the beginning Cheryl had been very jealous and possessive to the point of never letting Darren out of her sight. As more children came along it became more difficult, but Cheryl either followed Darren around or made his life hell when he returned. Darren ran a market stall and Cheryl insisted on sitting with him whenever she could. She always accompanied him to the wholesalers, going round with him while the children remained in the van. Whenever he went to the pub she turned up looking for him, the children in tow. They battled every minute of the day on every issue.

During counselling much came out about Cheryl's unhappy childhood and why she behaved as she did, but it didn't make a bit of difference to either of them. The counsellor could see that Darren had played his part in creating this difficult situation, but Darren himself was not able to recognise it. The only emotions they were able to acknowledge and express were ones of anger and bitterness. They were locked in a power struggle of resentment which began the moment they woke up and started to argue about who should give the children breakfast. Often the children would end up getting it for themselves.

After a time the counsellor stopped trying to help Cheryl and Darren to communicate and started instead on the way they behaved. In the first session of the new approach they talked about the morning row over feeding the children. What would help them resolve this? They both agreed they would have to get up at the same time. How would they manage that? They agreed that the only way they would be able to do it without either losing face was for both of them to put one foot on the floor at exactly the same moment, then swing round and put the other foot on the floor at the same time. At that session they also agreed who would put what on the kitchen table: Darren would get the cereal out of the cupboard, Cheryl the milk out of the fridge, and so on.

At the next session Darren and Cheryl reported with pleased surprise that this strange contract had worked. They'd stuck to what they said and hadn't found it difficult. Every day that week had got off to a good beginning and they were eager to approach other similar problems in the same way. Over the weeks they renegotiated their entire daily pattern.

The improvement was obvious and very cheering to Darren, Cheryl and the counsellor, who judged that it was now time to tackle Cheryl's possessiveness. Why would Cheryl never let Darren go to the wholesaler on his own? She feared that he would chat up one of the girl assistants. Their first task was for Cheryl to accompany Darren to the wholesaler, but instead of going round with him she would stand at a distance and watch how he behaved. Darren was to do nothing to make her jealous in the way he looked at other women. Later they tried Cheryl waiting in a nearby cafe while Darren shopped on his own. They progressed to the point where Cheryl would let Darren go to the wholesaler on his own, but he would come straight home every time – he wouldn't slip off somewhere with his mates unless he told her first.

By the time Cheryl felt able to do this and trust Darren her jealousy had almost disappeared and their entire relationship had improved. They were happy together for the first time since meeting. Then they surprised the counsellor. They had become so good and confident about negotiating that they came in one day with a radical plan of their own. For three days a week Cheryl was going to do her share of shopping at the wholesaler and running the market stall while Darren looked after the children. On the other three days Darren would carry out the work on his own while Cheryl stayed at home.

They came for a few more sessions before stopping counselling. Their family life had improved out of all recognition. Cheryl had developed more confidence since she had started working, and Darren had discovered how much he enjoyed being a stay-at-home father when it was his turn. By changing practical matters they had turned a destructive relationship into a happy, workable one.

DEALING WITH DIFFICULT EMOTIONS

We have already looked briefly at the problems of acknowledging and expressing difficult emotions. Now we need to look more closely at this

---

! ═══════════════ *Task* ═══════════════

Goodbyes and hellos

Have you got into the habit of giving each other a quick peck on greeting or parting, or barely noticing whether your partner has left or arrived?

Agree to take five minutes to do this properly at the beginning and end of a day. Concentrate your full attention on each other: touch, smile and be pleasant. If you know your partner is in for a hard day, let him or her know you'll be thinking about it.

!

> ═══════════════Talking point ═══════════════
>
> ### Let's pretend
>
> There is a true story about a married couple of American psychologists who were going through such a bad patch in their marriage that they were on the brink of divorcing.
>
> As a practical professional experiment they made a pact that for three months they would behave towards each other *as though* they were happily married, after which they would go ahead with divorce proceedings. But at the end of this time of behaving lovingly and respectfully towards each other their marriage had become happy again and they no longer thought of divorcing.
>
> Discuss this situation and why it should have made such a difference.

and particularly at two of the strongest and hardest to bear: jealousy and anger. All emotions are complicated and connected to other feelings, but these two are like the tops of volcanos and hide deeply buried feelings and memories from the past. Strong emotions such as these need closer examination because to deal with them it is often necessary to find out from where they come.

Strong emotions tend to burst forth or leak out in unhelpful ways when they become too much to bear. For most people it is frightening to look at such things closely. When you have strong negative feelings about your partner you resist examining them in case the relationship itself blows apart and leaves you with nothing. Many people fear being on their own. They will put up with a lot of hardship and misery in a relationship rather than confront the reasons for the problems and try to change them, afraid that doing so would cause them to break up.

As we saw earlier, everyone has some emotions they find easier to handle and express than others, and many people find it difficult when their partners are suffering certain emotions.

How well you talk about emotional matters is a good guide to the state of your relationship. As we have seen, avoiding them only works for a limited time. Life appears easier when they can be ignored. But strong emotions will surface again at some time and the more you are in the habit of avoiding them the harder to handle they become.

These are some points to bear in mind when emotions are strong:

- **Timing.** Because emotional matters are difficult to talk about many people wait until they are ready to explode before bringing them up. If you wait until 'the last straw', you are likely to be so emotional that you will have little control over what you say or do. Such confrontations become rows, or weepy scenes and are less likely to be resolved by useful solutions.

6————————Talking point————————

What happened next?

Read the following incidents and discuss what you think it is likely the people involved did next.

Carol and Michael were woken in the morning by their eight-year-old daughter Rachel bringing them a cup of tea she had made – the first time she had ever done this. Over breakfast they all had a laugh over something they heard on the news. At work, Carol's supervisor told her that she had recommended her for a pay rise. Carol's mother rang in the afternoon to say that Rachel, whom she collected from school, was excited by having been put in charge of part of the school garden. She was going to stay the night and look through granny's gardening books. Carol met a friend after work and they had a good chat about her friend's forthcoming wedding. Carol arrived home the same time as Michael, who told her that he had had an accident and although unhurt had put the car out of action. How do you think Carol reacted?

It was Martin's fortieth birthday. Sally, his wife, gave him a card which made jokes about his age – but he couldn't see the funny side. His train was late and his boss didn't believe his excuse. Later a younger man who had been with the firm a short time was promoted over him. On the way home he couldn't get a seat on the train and had to stand for two hours. Someone bashed his shin with a briefcase and Martin shouted at him. The man was rude back. When Martin got in Sally told him that she had booked a restaurant for his birthday treat, but she had had her bag stolen and was now without money or credit cards. How do you think Martin reacted?

When you imagined what Carol and Martin would have said or done in these situations, how much do you think the events of their days contributed to your decisions?

9

These are some examples of bad timing: the moment your partner walks through the door at the end of a day; at the end of any bad or difficult day; after you have had a row with someone else, or been at the receiving end of rudeness; when either of you is tired. Equally bad is the habit of choosing a time when you feel protected from your partner – usually when you are in public, with family or friends around. Although you might feel more able to express what you want to say when others are around, this is likely to make your partner feel defensive or angry and to embarrass the witnesses. Other people choose a moment when their partners are ill, sad or depressed, which also creates resentment and bad feeling.

Good timing is when you are relatively calm and when there is plenty of time to talk about the issue. This rarely happens without planning. Making a decision to talk matters through and agreeing on the day and time to do so is the best way.

● **Knowing what you really feel.** Planning a time to talk about these matters allows you to examine your feelings more calmly. During an explosion of jealousy, misery or anger it can be hard to recognise all the emotional factors that have led you to feel as you do. It is when you can see these for yourself that you are best able to tell your partner what the real problem is. For instance, jealousy over your partner's attention to someone else might be to do with a lack of self-confidence. It is easier to attack your partner by saying, 'You have no idea what a ridiculous spectacle you make of yourself behaving like that!' or 'You're so selfish – you have no consideration for my feelings!' than to admit, 'When I see you paying attention to someone else I feel unattractive and insecure and I feel like hurting you too.'

Expressing what you really feel is an act of courage. When you are part of a couple, it is easy to be afraid of saying what you need or want because of fear of what the other person might think. Telling how you really feel makes you vulnerable and requires trust. If both of you can do it then you will find yourselves growing closer, even if what you have been expressing is negative.

● **Finding the right way to tell your partner.** When expressing what you feel it is important to do so in a way that your partner is *able* to listen to. Angry, blaming, punishing, hysterical, or over emotional tones will cause most listeners to switch off or become defensive. The calmer you are the easier you are to listen to.

In the same way, expressing what you feel by attacking your partner confuses your message. The issue is how *you* are feeling. It is those negative feelings that need to change and by explaining fully and honestly what they are your partner has the necessary information to make changes in how he or she behaves – you can't *force* a change. Usually you both need to make changes – to compromise – and to know how to do so both of you need to be honest about your own feelings.

If what you say comes as a complete surprise or shock to your partner, you must also be prepared to explain what you feel more than once. An important announcement about your feelings, if it comes out of the blue, can easily be dismissed as 'just a mood'. One counsellor says that certain fundamental, difficult issues might have to be explained over a period of many sessions of talking together before your partner fully takes them in. This is different from nagging: you are making the effort to clarify your own feelings, not attempting to change your partner's ideas or beaviour. In counselling one person will often cry 'But I told you that!' when the other has no memory of something that was clearly important. Having got it off his or her chest once, the first partner often feels that it need never be mentioned again – and then suffers from the fact that talking about it has apparently made no difference.

● **Making assumptions.** Good and positive changes can only come about when you do talk freely and openly to each other about your feelings. What often happens is that you don't talk about the things that matter most to you.

When you don't talk, two things happen. The first is that you make assumptions about what each other thinks and feels; you look at how your partner behaves and perhaps misinterpret it. The other unfortunate result is that you assume that your partner should know how you feel deep inside. This means that you either believe that your partner is purposely behaving in ways to upset you, or, if your partner is obviously unaware of how you feel, you think it means he or she doesn't love you enough.

An example of how assumptions can affect a relationship is shown by Lucy, who came for counselling on her own soon after her fortieth birthday. Mark, her husband, was forty-one, and they had a son of seventeen. Part of Lucy's problem was that turning forty had stirred up a lot of dissatisfaction in her. It had caused her to look at her life – and she didn't like what she saw. She and Mark both had good jobs, all the money they needed and a lovely lifestyle. For Lucy this wasn't enough. She wanted to feel excited and purposeful – that life began at forty – but instead she felt that it just meant a slow decline. Mark on the other hand, she said, was smug and self-satisfied. He was content with the life they had built and felt none of her restless need for 'something else'. There was little particularly wrong with the marriage but Lucy felt there was nothing in it for her.

Mark was upset by Lucy's sudden rejection of him and couldn't understand why counselling should be necessary. Nevertheless, he agreed to accompany Lucy to her second session. The counsellor says, 'He was so terrified that he could neither move nor speak – and he never came again.' Despite this, Lucy continued to come, and reported that Mark was willing to talk about the sessions and participate in what she had gathered at home.

Much of the counselling was involved with examining Lucy's early life and relationship with her parents. There were factors here that had affected Lucy's confidence and as these were looked at and dealt with Lucy began to feel very much better about herself. As she did so, she said that her relationship with Mark started to improve. Even so, Lucy still maintained that Mark's satisfaction with their steady and boring life made her see little future in the relationship.

The turning point came when the counsellor said to Lucy, 'You keep telling me how smug and self-satisfied Mark is, but you have never given me any evidence of it. Have you asked him how he feels or explained your own dissatisfaction?'

The next session saw Lucy transformed. During the week she had sat down with Mark and told him everything she felt. She asked how he felt about the way they were going. He revealed that he had been dissatisfied with his work. He had ideas about what he wanted to do instead, but it would mean an initial drop in income and moving to another city. He hadn't mentioned this because Lucy seemed so settled.

Both of them wanted change and challenge but neither had mentioned it because they assumed the other was content. By the time Lucy saw the counsellor they had put their house on the market and Mark was making the first moves to set himself up in his new job. Lucy was finding out about getting a transfer and felt rejuvenated and excited by this new phase in their marriage.

Jealousy

Jealousy makes you behave in ways that can harm your relationship and make the jealous feelings even stronger. Unless you are able to understand the reasons and feelings that contribute to making you feel extreme jealousy you are unable to change the situation. Beverley is an example of someone who suffered the torments of jealousy for many years before counselling helped her and her husband Jack make the necessary changes to improve their relationship.

Beverley, a sad, quiet, overweight woman, came for counselling on her own. Jack, in common with quite a number of men, didn't feel able to face counselling but was happy for Beverley to attend and to discuss matters with him afterwards.

The story Beverley came with was that Jack had had an affair some years before. The woman was the wife in a couple with whom they had been friendly and had often accompanied on outings as a foursome. Beverley had always found the friendship difficult. She felt left out by the other three on their evenings together. Eventually when she discovered about the affair, she and Jack had moved away and she felt that they had put it behind them. Now, however, it seemed that the pattern was repeating itself. They had made friends with another couple they saw regularly and Beverley again felt miserable and left out by the other three and was convinced that Jack was having an affair with the wife.

One of the first things the counsellor discussed with Beverley was her feeling of exclusion. What were her first memories of having felt like this? Beverley, it turned out, was the adopted child of a couple who could not have children. Her adoptive father had died and her mother had married again and this time had two children of her own. Beverley's stepfather had never liked her and her mother seemed more attached to the younger children. Sometimes they would go on holiday and leave her with her grandmother, her adoptive father's mother. She had always felt the odd one out. Feeling excluded was for Beverley the most painful of all emotions.

As this emerged in counselling Beverley saw that she tended to overreact to any situation that made her feel as she had done in the past. She began to see that the strength of her feelings often bore little relation to what was actually happening. She imagined that people were leaving her out even if this was not the case. Then she told the counsellor that she thought that perhaps Jack, too, had felt excluded by his family. Jack came from a well-educated family, all of whom were lawyers. He had not been academically bright and had become a skilled carpenter, working for a large building firm. He had little in common with the rest of his family, who patronised him.

When Beverley talked to Jack about her theory he was very struck by the truth of it: he had felt lonely and excluded throughout his childhood and later. He was so intrigued by what this might mean that he agreed to join Beverely for the counselling.

Now the counsellor gained an even clearer picture of Beverley and Jack's life together. The two loners had originally been attracted to each other because of these feelings they had in common, though they were not aware of it. They both found company threatening, but they handled this in different ways. Jack acted up. He became very loud and exuberant and would try to make people like him by telling jokes and being the life and soul of the party. Beverley was the reverse. She would sit in a corner and become quieter and quieter. The louder Jack got the more panicked she felt. When they came home after an evening out she would harangue him and put him down for his stupid, loutish behaviour and accuse him of paying too much attention to other women. During their entire marriage she had suffered from jealousy – convinced that popular Jack would run off with someone else. His affair had confirmed her fears. Since then her jealousy had become worse. Jack was not, in fact, having an affair now and had no desire to, but Beverley was constantly on at him about his shortcomings and his pathetic interest in other women. In public she was sullen and bad-tempered, eaten with jealous feelings.

Now that they had both pinpointed their behaviour as resulting from their feelings of exclusion, the counsellor worked with them on how they could change matters. They agreed on a number of ways of doing this, but the most important concerned their social life, which caused most of the problems. Beverley agreed that she would do nothing to squash Jack's social exuberance or make him feel bad about himself, and he would make sure that she was included in the fun and not allowed to feel left out.

It was hard for them to change some of their habits of behaviour and they came for many more sessions until they that felt they had got it right. But the counsellor says that every time she saw them after this they looked better and happier. When they were no longer doing things that distressed each other they started to feel better about themselves. As they liked themselves more so they liked each other more. Beverley joined a slimming club and lost two stone. Now that Jack was making her feel more wanted she felt the urge to do something about the way she looked. Jack felt more confident in himself now that Beverley had stopped putting him down. He persuaded a local financier to put money into setting him up as a quality furniture maker on his own.

Jack was proud of the way Beverley looked and the way she was now blossoming in company – he could see that giving her more attention stopped her resentful feelings. Beverley no longer believed Jack was having an affair and could understand that by putting him down she had pushed him into ever more flamboyant behaviour to prove how much other people liked him. Beverley was proud of his new business; she had never rated his work highly before. The counsellor says, 'They looked different people. They valued themselves and each other. Every time they came in they looked younger and happier.'

Natural jealousy

It was natural for Beverley to feel jealous when Jack had his affair, and it is natural to find it difficult to regain feelings of trust after an affair. Jealousy and possessiveness can continue for months after the end of an affair and it can take a long time to rebuild trust. Sometimes it is never totally rebuilt – but there is enough for the couple to live happily yet differently together. This is looked at in more detail in the section on affairs in the next chapter.

It is also natural to feel pangs of jealousy over other specific incidents – your partner's obvious admiration for someone else, for instance. But in a healthy relationship these feelings pass, either because you talk them through or because you are able to put them in proportion.

Beverley's jealousy went beyond any obvious causes. She had always felt it, even before there was a reason, and she had created a situation that made Jack's behaviour worse and intensified her own pain. The jealousy we are looking at here is the extreme and irrational kind that has more to do with the feelings of the person experiencing it than the actions of the partner.

Is jealousy a sign of love?

Jealous feelings are usually at their strongest when you are newly in love and do not yet feel secure in your partner's affection. When you are at the stage of being intoxicated by your partner's 'perfection' it is common to believe that other people must feel as you do and that your luck in catching such a paragon might not last.

Jealousy is a part of early love and it can be very flattering when your partner seems constantly on edge at the thought of losing you. Jealousy in the early stages is like an aphrodisiac: it makes you feel passionate, you want to be close to your partner, to make love, in order to reaffirm that you yourself are wanted and loved. Happy couples in the early stages sometimes play the slightly dangerous game of flirting with other people precisely for this reason. Jealousy and possessiveness are normal features of adolescent relationships.

As jealousy is so much a part of early love, at the beginning it is often welcomed. But this changes when the relationship settles down. Once you stop being wrapped up in each other, constant togetherness and the exclusion of other people become inappropriate. A good settled relationship needs both partners to have a certain amount of independence and separateness. Jealousy that continues to figure strongly no longer feels like love: instead it is suffocating, controlling, and suggests a lack of trust in the partner and the relationship. The jealousy that once brought the couple together now starts to create difficulties.

The main reasons behind irrational jealousy

Irrationally destructive jealousy has three main causes, which are very similar and are interconnected:

- **Lack of confidence.** If you lack confidence in yourself then you also find it difficult to believe that someone can truly love you. Some very successful and apparently confident people have deep-down doubts about their own lovableness, which usually go back to early childhood experiences. When these have had a profound effect on you it can be difficult to trust the words and actions even of people who are obviously deeply in love with you. Somewhere inside you believe that it can't last. You are alert to every real or imagined incident that proves your partner's love is fading.

● **Fear of change.** Excessive jealousy first becomes noticeable when the nature of a relationship starts to change and settle down, becoming less romantic. But irrational jealousy can also be triggered by other changes, perhaps later in a relationship. People who subconsciously fear that change must always be for the worse, or that it means a rejection of the earlier relationship rather than a natural move into something different, will react by becoming jealous and possessive.

When one partner's needs within a relationship change the other can feel threatened and as a consequence hangs on tighter than ever, afraid that change might mean the end. In a good relationship each of you develops your own life, thereby building your own sense of inner security, which has the effect of strengthening the relationship. If your sense of security is based entirely upon your partner and the relationship, this can make you frightened and dependent, which weakens the ties between you.

One counsellor notices that it is often when one partner is making obvious changes and developing in new ways that the other reacts by becoming jealous. She has seen many cases of women in their late twenties or early thirties who feel restricted and tied down by the needs of the family become irrationally jealous when their husbands' careers are taking off and their lives seem to be opening out. Men, she has found, often react like this later on, perhaps when the children have grown up and their wives have made the decision to go back to work while they themselves are in the same old jobs. The changes in their wives make the men insecure and possessive.

● **Fear of being alone.** This is clearly linked to the other two, though not every irrationally jealous person has this fear; some go the other way and avoid the pain of being left by choosing to be alone. Like Beverley, this can develop because you felt excluded in some way as a child and the fear and misery you felt then can stay with you in later life. Sometimes it is too far back for you to remember, perhaps you were ill as a baby and were separated from your mother. If something affected your closest early relationship you can grow up feeling bad about yourself and with a need to have someone close at all costs. Other later difficulties

– with best friends at school, for instance – can add to your feelings of insecurity.

Fears of being alone can also develop if you come from a family that has broken down through separation, divorce or death. This experience can leave you with the subconscious feeling that you can't trust a partner to stay around and a general lack of confidence in your ability to maintain a relationship.

The vicious circle of jealousy

Jealousy makes you behave in ways that are destructive to your relationship and even when you know that you are doing this it can be hard to stop. Behind the jealousy lurks the expectation that your relationship is bound to fail. By behaving destructively you are making sure that it *does* fail. But the more destructive you are and the worse your relationship becomes the more jealous and insecure you feel.

You have to be able to recognise the part you are playing in the vicious circle before you can do something positive to change it. These are some of the common ways that jealous behaviour can eat away at your relationship, destroying the good in it:

● **Trying to control.** When you fear that your partner is being unfaithful – or that he or she will be unfaithful if you don't watch out – you will usually try to control every aspect of your partner's life. You feel the need to keep tabs on your partner all the time. You want to be together constantly, and when you can't, you need to know exactly what your partner has been up to. A typical example of this is the young wife who needed to know what her husband was doing every minute of the day. If he went out for lunch with colleagues from work she would want to know exactly what had happened: who was sitting next to him and what was said. He took to pretending that he never sat next to a female colleague because if he told his wife he had she would fly into a jealous rage that lasted for hours.

What usually accompanies this behaviour is an unwillingness to believe what your partner tells you. You will try to catch your partner out by looking through diaries, clothing and private drawers. One woman noted down the number of the nearest telephone box, convinced that whenever her husband took the dog for a walk he would be phoning his mistress. She would call the number herself, and if it was engaged she would rush out of the house to try to catch her husband using the telephone.

● **Punishing.** Controlling behaviour is quite obviously the result of jealousy, and some people also act out their jealous feelings by punishing

❝─────────────── Talking point ═══════════

Patterns

Within counselling sessions counsellors sometimes ask people to show their relationships symbolically, using coins or stones to represent the people in their lives and their relationships with each other. For example, one woman used a penny coin to represent herself and surrounded it with ten-pence pieces to represent her children, her sisters and her best friend. For her husband she chose a fifty-pence coin which she placed outside the circle. At another session a man represented himself as a pound coin and piled the other coins representing his family on top of it. Another man who was married yet had had many affairs and one-night stands, simply picked up the coins and scattered them on the table, saying that it had no meaning.

There is no right or wrong way to do this, and only the person doing the arranging knows what it means. The counsellor will ask, 'How does that person feel?' pointing to one of the coins, or say, 'If you could change the arrangement what would you change it to and why?'

This is a difficult task to do for yourself as the trained counsellor helps you bring up the relevant points usefully but you can try if you want. Discuss with your partner the three examples given above and say what you think these people might be feeling about their relationships.

❞

and being aggressive. Very often the partner has no idea that this behaviour springs from jealousy and is hurt and angered by it.

This can take various forms. One of the most common is putting your partner down, as Beverley did to Jack. Because you yourself are feeling unconfident you want to take away your partner's confidence as well and make him or her feel as bad as you do. If, as many people do, you make a good job of hiding your lack of confidence by boasting or behaving arrogantly your partner will be even more demoralised by your behaviour and will be more likely to respond by being unpleasant back. This, of course, will reduce your confidence further and make your jealous feelings worse.

Another way of punishing and hiding your jealousy at the same time is to behave sulkily or angrily to your partner but not explain why. Your bad mood can cause you to pick on your partner for a variety of reasons, causing rows between you which never even touch on the real problem. It can also take the form of refusing sex – even though you fear this will send your partner into the arms of someone else – or of not showing love and affection in other ways. When you fear you are unlovable, deliberately making yourself so by bad behaviour feels 'right' even though it is making you and your partner unhappy.

● **Imagining.** This is when you indulge your jealous fears by making yourself imagine what your partner might be up to. You pick up on tiny clues such as your partner's momentary daydream or glance at someone else, and turn them into a full-scale drama in your mind in which you imagine you know precisely what your partner is thinking or doing behind your back.

This is sometimes accompanied by physical feelings of sickness. Your imaginings lead you to become full of overwhelming anxiety. One counsellor had a client who made herself ill with jealousy. Her partner only had to look at someone else for her to be physically sick.

● **Paying back.** Vivid imaginings caused by jealous feelings can lead some people to want to pay their partners back by indulging in open and obvious flirtation or even by having a revenge affair. One man started an affair with his secretary shortly after his wife returned to work for just this reason. He couldn't believe his innocent wife simply wanted a job to occupy her hours, and became convinced that she was carrying on with a number of men – his affair was to show her that he could do the same.

● **Ending the relationship.** Some jealous people find waiting for what they believe to be the inevitable end so unbearable that they decide to end the relationship themselves. When the relationship hits a snag they become so sure it means the end of love that they haven't any incentive to try to work through the problem. Sometimes they will do this because their own imaginings have become so real and troublesome that they see problems even where there are none. One woman left her husband after she saw him talking to a male friend at a party. She said that she could 'tell by the expression' on the other man's face that her husband was confessing to an affair, and she refused to believe her husband or his friend that this was not so.

What jealousy does to your relationship

Prolonged and excessive irrational jealousy can only harm a relationship. The form the damage takes varies, but a relationship is never improved by the jealous feelings and actions of one of the partners.

Sometimes the partner who has been accused of infidelity will, in the end, become unfaithful. As one woman said, 'I was being punished for something I hadn't done so I thought I might as well do it.' Or the partner who is being too controlled might leave the relationship because the pressure has become unbearable.

Some couples stay together despite the jealousy but do so unhappily. The 'marital fit' might be one where the jealousy is part of the glue that keeps a couple together. While hating the actions of the jealous partner, the other might need the safety of the relationship however unpleasant it has become – which was how Jack felt before he and Beverley went for counselling.

Sex often becomes a problem because of the bad feelings that jealousy creates in both partners. As we have seen, at the beginning of a relationship jealousy can increase passion, and it can do so (if only temporarily) later on. But the more tense and unbalanced the relationship becomes the more jealousy will sour the sexual side too.

Coping with jealousy

Curing yourself of jealousy is not easy to do, particularly if the reasons for it are rooted in the long-forgotten past. It can be hard to work out for yourself why you feel as you do, especially if you are convinced that it is your partner's fault. Counselling is usually the best way to sort out the rational feelings from the irrational ones and to find a way to come to terms with childhood reasons behind your jealousy. Counselling can also help you to feel better about yourself and use these new feelings to combat jealousy.

Nevertheless, if you recognise that your jealousy is harming your relationship it is possible to take some steps on your own without counselling, in order to help yourself feel better and improve matters between you.

● **Think twice.** If you are able to see that you have formed the habit of behaving in some of the ways listed above, then you have the opportunity to change them, although this is easier said than done when you are in the grip of strong, painful jealousy. The first step is to notice when you are about to act unhelpfully and think about what you are doing. Remember what effect your actions will have on yourself and your partner and how they are likely to make matters worse for you.

Over time you might find that you are able to stop yourself behaving in some of the more destructive ways. Catching yourself when you start to imagine the worst is also helpful. Find something else to occupy you and make a deliberate effort to switch your mind to another topic.

● **Examine your feelings.** See how far back you can trace your feelings of jealousy. Try to remember times of misery in your childhood and see if they were to do with being lonely or the absence of a loved one. Remembering these feelings can help you to realise that what you feel now is connected to past experiences which sometimes cause you to overreact.

Looking at all the emotions connected to your jealousy is also useful. If you are in the habit of trying to control your partner, you might also notice that you are feeling fear and panic. If you punish your partner, think of the sad and angry feelings that are leading you to do this. When you have a better idea of why you behave as you do it is helpful to explain these other emotions and motives to your partner at moments when you are feeling calmer and more trusting. Explaining the fears that made you fly into a jealous rage, for example, or the anxiety that drove you to make your partner feel worthless is helpful to both of you. Bringing these thoughts out into the open can make you feel more rational about them. It also allows your partner to understand what is happening. Accusing your partner of having an affair puts him or her on the defensive, whereas saying 'When you come home late I find myself thinking you must be having an affair,' gives your partner the opportunity to reassure you or to change the aspects of his or her behaviour that are causing problems.

• **Develop your independence.** The less you rely on your partner the better you will feel about yourself. Developing confidence and feelings of self-worth is the best way to cure excessive jealousy. There is little that your partner can do to reassure you that you are valued until you learn to value yourself.

These positive feelings can be built quite deliberately by developing your independence. This means putting effort into other friendships outside your relationship, perhaps finding a job or hobby that interests you or for which you have a talent, returning to education, or training for a more challenging career. When you develop a sense of yourself as having worth separate from your relationship it is easier to tolerate separateness from your partner.

• **Pamper yourself.** This is also to do with developing confidence. Show yourself that you value yourself by doing things that you enjoy. Counsellors find that jealous people have low self-esteem and often feel they have no right to consider their own needs. They will encourage people who suffer from jealousy to do something just for themselves, such as taking up a sport if that appeals, or buying something affordable for a treat.

• **Understanding separateness.** Side by side with developing your own confidence and separate life goes the understanding that your partner deserves this too. Possessiveness, when it is damaging, leads to feelings of ownership: you think your partner should belong to you entirely, and should have no independent life. You feel unable to share the other person. But you can never own another human being, partner, child or friend. There is nothing practical that you can do to make yourself accept this fact, but acknowledging that is true will help you in the long run.

Tell yourself you do not own your partner, however uncomfortable that thought makes you feel. What you can do is strive to make the relationship something that is worth wanting for itself. The more you come to believe this the more motivated you will be to stop behaving in ways that make the relationship unpleasant.

• **Learn to trust.** This is another thing that is very much easier said than done. Trust is the direct opposite of control and people who feel trusted usually want to repay that trust by acting in a trustworthy way.

Trust does not mean a blind belief that your partner will never stray or act in ways that you would not like, but it does entail creating a distance between you. A distance based on trust is, surprisingly, one that makes partners feel closer and more happily relaxed with each other.

While you can't force yourself to feel trust, you can start to behave in trusting ways and see what effect this has on your relationship. That would involve not insisting on a blow-by-blow account of your partner's day, for instance, and resisting the temptation to go through your partner's personal things for 'evidence'. It would also involve accepting your partner's word without interrogation or a show of disbelief, even if you feel it in your heart. It would mean one by one letting go of any controlling habits you have developed and seeing whether by doing so matters improve. If this is accompanied by your explanations of why you behave in irrationally jealous ways you might be pleasantly surprised at how your partner starts to take your feelings into account.

• **Living with a jealous partner.** If your partner is excessively jealous then there are a number of ways you can help matters. Firstly make the effort to listen to what your partner is saying about the way he or she feels, particularly if this includes an honest expression of deep and painful feelings.

You must understand the lack of confidence behind possessive behaviour and the ways in which you contribute to this. If you know your partner's jealousy is irrational, you need to do more than say, 'I'm not doing any of the things you're accusing me of – get off my back!' You must find out if there are simple things you can do to reassure your partner, such as telephoning when you say you will. If your partner is upset by the attention you pay to other people at parties, you can make sure you spend some time with him or her, perhaps give the occasional hug or a smile across the room.

Most importantly, you need to help build your partner's confidence. In counselling, someone in your situation is encouraged to tell your partner what it is you love and like about him or her, and to continue to do this outside the sessions when you are at home. Although initially this seems contrived it eventually becomes a habit and feels natural. Think of ways of making your partner feel 'good enough'; make sure that you spend time together – going out or making special efforts to talk when you are at home.

Getting the balance right

A degree of possessiveness and togetherness is healthy in a relationship, and when it is positive it has its warm side. You need to feel that your partner cares what you are doing, that it *does* matter whether you are faithful or not.

Caring what your partner does is natural, but the constant anxiety of always wondering what he or she is up to is not. You need to feel independent, yet part of a relationship. For example, if your partner is going to be late home it is normal to like to be told so that you can plan your evening. That is not possessive or controlling. It involves care on both sides: one caring and showing enough respect to want to let the partner know, the other caring enough to worry if the partner is late.

Anger

The question people ask themselves is, 'If this is love, why do I feel so angry?' One of the myths of romantic love is that if two people are right for each other they will live in perfect harmony. It can be quite frightening to find yourself fighting with the one you love best and feeling anger, misery and sometimes dislike. Some couples hold off from fighting for many years, sure that heated disagreements are a sign that something is wrong between them and therefore keep the peace at all costs.

But thinking differently from someone is part of being an individual, as we have already seen, and anger is a perfectly normal human emotion. A couple in a healthy, developing relationship are bound to clash from time to time. Ignoring angry feelings is more dangerous than expressing them. It is how you deal with them that counts. Proper handling of these emotions will make your relationship even better.

!————————————— *Task* —————— ——————

The hit list

If you are constantly being made angry by your partner and your relationship it can be hard to know what to do about it. One way is to sort out what makes you feel angry and why it does so.

Keep a diary of your angry moments. Note down the incidents that triggered them off. Underneath write down what else you were feeling at the same time. This can include physical feelings, such as tiredness, headache or other pain, but it is even more important to note other emotions. These are some common underlying feelings:

sadness	envy	nervous-	depression
fear	jealousy	ness	self-dislike
guilt	insecurity	hurt pride	protective-
		grief	ness

Once you have a better idea of the other feelings involved you can start to sort out what you and your partner can do to acknowledge and deal with those feelings and therefore begin to remove the causes for your constant anger.

!

What anger means

Anger has gained itself a bad reputation as a negative emotion. It is thought to be emotional poison, destructive of a happy relationship. In fact, anger is just a warning flag, a sign that an issue that needs proper attention is being touched upon. Anger is the most accurate pointer to what is important to you.

Calling the passionate collection of emotions you feel 'anger' is a little misleading. It is not one single, pure emotion. Anger is generated by other feelings. Think of what you would feel if you saw someone hitting an old lady; next imagine hearing that your partner is having an affair; then picture being passed over for a promotion you knew you deserved. All these situations are likely to make you feel angry, but the underlying emotions that boiled into anger are different in each case. This is partly why anger is so difficult to handle properly. Anger can be so powerful, making you blind and deaf with rage, that it is hard to remain in touch with the feelings that generated it. This is particularly so in a relationship, where the causes may not be obvious even to you – anger triggered off by an incident that stirs up difficult emotions connected to something that upset you long ago. But the key to dealing with the anger – really curing it rather than trying to suppress it – means understanding the feelings that gave rise to it and then taking steps to change the situations that trigger off those feelings.

Expressing anger

If anger is so normal and holding it in is wrong, then presumably there is nothing wrong with showing it as and when you feel it? This is true – but only to a certain extent. Strong anger makes you reckless, stops you thinking rationally, and can make you hit out verbally and sometimes physically too. Anger makes you want to attack, hurt, and win.

The trouble is that letting your anger dictate what you do and say only affects your immediate feelings, the angry ones, and anger invites attack in its turn. Really letting rip at your partner can feel right and good at that moment. It may also make you feel a little better: allowing angry feelings full expression often allows them to evaporate. After all that noise and fury you don't feel so angry any more.

But while the heat is taken out of the moment the other feelings that led to the anger remain completely unsatisfied. They may not bother you for the moment, but they don't go away. Having a 'good row' can sometimes make it even more difficult to show or deal with these feelings. In anger you are strong, but the feelings that gave rise to the anger may be ones of weakness and fear. When you are scoring points off your partner, showing how clever with words you are, how strong and uncaring you can appear it becomes very hard to acknowledge, even to yourself, that what lies behind all this is, for instance, fear that you have lost your partner's love.

Connie and Dan are a good example of a couple who had developed an unproductive cycle of rows that momentarily made them feel better, but which ultimately left their problem untouched.

The relationship was in shreds when they started counselling. They would argue viciously in the counselling room, both punishing each other with hurtful remarks, and there was no apparent warmth in their marriage. When they rowed at home Dan would become physically violent. They were staying together for the sake of the children, and it seemed as though they hoped the counsellor would act as referee and take sides and decide once and for all who was right.

Connie had the kind of unhappy background that left her resistant to love and affection. She had been let down often and she had reacted by deciding that no one would ever be allowed to get close to her. Intimacy embarrassed her, and she had developed an uncaring manner in case she was ever left alone.

Dan had different problems. He'd been given a lot of responsibility when young – his father had left when he was eleven and his duties had been to take his father's place in his mother's life and be in charge of his younger brother. He blamed himself for the fact that his mother was unhappy and he felt guilty about the times he had disciplined his brother. He was left with the feeling that he was no good to other people and consequently was afraid to get close to them. He had developed a blustering manner. 'Tell people what you think of them first' was his motto: let them know you don't like them before you find out that they don't like you.

The pattern in their marriage was as follows. Dan would become enraged by Connie's coolness. He had a fiery temper and this would become uncontrollable. He would keep on at Connie until he had some reaction, taking every opportunity to bully, needle, and patronise her. When she tried to get away from him he would trail around after her, sticking the verbal knife in. Finally she would become demented with anger and attack in her turn. She would tell Dan that the kids loathed and feared him before she withdrew into icy misery. Days of Connie sulking would follow.

At this point Dan would feel terrible. Feeling lonely and guilty he would try to make up. He would wheedle, buy Connie flowers or do something else special for her. Reluctantly she would allow herself to be wooed, to be made love to. For two or three days Dan would feel good about how he was behaving to his wife.

Then Connie would start. She would make a caustic comment about the loving gestures Dan had made. She might say, 'Of course you only bought the flowers because you feel so guilty about the fact that you are a monster.' Dan would be hurt and disappointed, and soon became angry, this would result in Connie becoming cool and withdrawn again. Dan's anger would increase, he would panic at her untouchable remoteness and they would be back at the beginning of the violent vicious circle.

The counsellor helped them to see what was happening. They were both incapable of showing each other positive feelings until they were exhausted by the power of their negative feelings. They never said anything nice to each other and both had difficulty showing affection.

During counselling they learnt to praise each other when appropriate and to treat each other with more respect. They found this difficult – thought it almost stupid – to begin with. Then Connie began to listen to Dan and understand how isolated he felt from the family and how this hurt him. When she understood how she contributed to his anger she became softer and he reacted by gaining more control of his temper. They began to recognise that when they were nice to each other the constant prickle of irritation they both felt went – and with it the follow-on of the more violent feelings of anger. As they made the difficult transition to looking for things to value rather than attack in each other they started to feel better about themselves – and once that happened they were able to be pleasant to each other more freely.

When the pattern was first broken Dan became depressed. He said that he missed the rows – at least they made up and had a few good days together before it started all over again. But as the relationship continued to improve neither of them had any wish to return to the old pattern. Both of them had feared showing soft, vulnerable, loving feelings and had only been able to do so when extreme anger had collapsed into misery. Now that they felt more trusting and able to develop their loving feelings without the framework of anger, every area of their life together was happier.

Avoiding anger

Many people put a lot of effort into keeping angry feelings at bay in a relationship. There is a lot to be said for keeping the peace, but not if it means choking down thoughts and feelings. A peace that is negotiated after angry feelings are expressed and understood is more likely to last. A peace that is the result of repression is likely to make you feel unhappy, dissatisfied and depressed; it is like an armed truce that can end at any time.

Relationships without anger

When you are very much in love at the beginning of a relationship you are likely to find yourselves pretty much in agreement most of the time. You may even believe that this can continue for ever. But early love, as we have seen, is a powerful drug: under its influence you may not even notice your own much weaker (at that time) feelings of dissent, irritability or anger.

For some couples this peaceful existence endures and they find that they think the same way about most things. Neither finds anything about the other irritating, and instead respects the personality and views of his or her partner. Couples like this are usually quite calm people anyway, slow to anger and more generally tolerant. After all, two people can be very much in love and think alike about most matters but be hot-tempered and argue a lot of the time.

Other people also maintain happily peaceful relationships together because they have a strong and similar sense of humour, which surfaces to break the tension at crucial moments – rather than have a row they have a laugh.

For the majority of people, however, a relationship that is calm and relatively anger-free has to be worked at. They have made the decision that arguing passionately is counterproductive. They may find themselves disagreeing – even seriously – but they have found ways of dealing with these times without destructive anger. This approach is dealt with later in the section on helpful ways to argue.

Fear of anger

Many people avoid expressing anger because they are frightened by it: sometimes they will do anything to placate their partners and avoid being the target of anger. Some people live apparently quiet and peaceful lives together because they fear arguing: perhaps another person's aggression seems frightening, or their own angry feelings are so powerful that they are not sure that they can control them.

When only one of you shows anger it does not mean the other does not feel it. One partner can be liberated by shouting and rowing; but if the other is frightened, he or she might not respond. The shouter believes the air is being cleared, whereas in fact the silent partner is burying anger and hurt deeper and deeper.

One sure sign of this is whether either of you sulk. Sulking is a silent expression of anger, the main difference being that sulking gives no chance for the issue to be resolved.

In an unequal relationship, where you are not secure in your partner's love, you might try harder than ever to swallow your anger and not disagree with your partner for fear of losing whatever love. there is. If you are making great efforts to control your anger, which in itself makes you sad and depressed, you can be unaware of the contribution you are making to the unhappiness of your relationship.

Counselling can help by providing a safe place for you to experience and express angry feelings with an outsider who can see that there is fair play. Couples who learn during counselling that disagreeing is not the end of the world find they are more able to express anger naturally the rest of the time.

Anger in your past

If you find expressing anger or being on the receiving end of angry feelings frightening then the clue to why this could be usually lies somewhere in your past.

Your experience of anger when you were a child has a lot to do with it. How anger was dealt with within your family and how that made you feel will often dictate how you deal with anger later.

In some families anger is freely and frequently expressed. This can be frightening to little children, who never know when it is going to descend on them or what the consequences will be. Children from these families can grow up trying to avoid rows at all costs – or they can feel the urge to reproduce the pattern in their own adult relationships. Other children come from apparently peaceful homes, where there were tense undercurrents of anger or unhappiness. This can be equally frightening to the children, who grow up sensing these unspoken feelings and fearful of the unknown catastrophe that could happen if they were to be unleashed. If you have never experienced the healthy give-and-take of friendly arguing, the mere prospect of a raised voice can make you fear that it means the end of a relationship.

Couples with opposing attitudes to anger can find themselves with a communication problem. One might feel ready and able to express anger, but the other withdraws in fear – which increases the anger felt on both sides. Equally, if you are both afraid of expressing anger communication becomes difficult because you are unable to share an entire area of thoughts and feelings.

What happens to repressed anger

Breakdown of communication is the most obvious effect of repressed anger. You cannot communicate easily and freely if you have something important you are hiding. The cost of keeping anger inside is that it stifles the good feelings. This rots the fabric of a relationship – and an area in which this often shows is sex.

One counsellor gives the example of a man who came to see her alone, saying that after several years of marriage he was now impotent and he wanted sexual therapy to help him solve the problem. Relate, however, never refers couples or individuals for sexual therapy until they have looked closely at the rest of the relationship to see if there are any other problems. Communication between a couple needs to be as good as possible before sexual therapy starts.

In the case of this man it turned out that the onset of his impotency had coincided with his wife having an affair. He dismissed the fact very quickly and said, 'But I've forgiven her that, it's all over.' The counsellor knew that such an important event in a relationship could not be dismissed so casually, but the more she tried to get him to talk about his feelings connected to the affair the more resistant he became. Eventually he stopped coming for counselling – he seemed to think that if he allowed himself to acknowledge how angry he felt then the marriage might fall apart.

The reverse is often the case. During counselling, when couples are encouraged to come right out and say what they feel or want more assertively the feelings are released. Once you've expressed the anger you can let it go: it's not there clogging up everything else. And when that happens you feel very much closer sexually too.

Good anger and bad anger

People who find difficulty in expressing anger are often held up by the fact that they think anger is somehow bad. The emotion itself, however, is neutral. Anger becomes good or bad depending on how you use it. Someone who expresses anger freely is no better than the person who keeps it in if the anger is used destructively and punishingly.

Dealing properly with anger means not denying the feelings, but not letting them take you over either. Anger is 'bad' when you use it to attack or blame your partner, rather than whatever it is your partner is doing. 'Good' anger is expressed cleanly in terms of how you are feeling. It explains what aspect of the other's behaviour disturbs you but it doesn't judge or condemn the person concerned.

These points are looked at in more detail under helpful and unhelpful ways to argue.

ARGUING

The value of disagreements

Disagreements are natural and they are also useful. Even very similar people have their differences, and these are bound to come up when you live together. Part of a developing relationship is acknowledging the separateness and individuality of your partner, and disagreements serve to show you in what ways you are different. Frankly expressing what you feel and respecting your partner's right to have different ideas and emotions both contribute to your good feelings about your relationship. Some differences are more surprising or disturbing than others, but bringing them out into the open and coming to accept them increases your tolerance – another vital ingredient in a good relationship.

Sometimes a problem crops up or a decision needs to be made about which you feel passionately at odds with each other. If you have a good and tolerant relationship and have become used to listening and adjusting to each other's point of view you can eventually put all your negotiating skills to work. Practice will bring home to you the truth that more important than individual points of view is the wellbeing of the relationship – which often means both of you being prepared to give up something so that you can meet in the middle.

Flare ups

Occasional unimportant rows are very much a part of everyday living. Sometimes your day has gone badly and left you in an irritated state. You might be snappy and out-of-sorts and the least thing will get you going. If your partner has had a good day the row might not get very far, but if both of you are on edge you can end up scrapping over minor irritations or disagreements. These kind of rows leave you wondering next morning (or even an hour later) what they were all about, and you might feel silly and sorry. This happens to everyone and is not worth worrying over. You still need to fight by the rules however, or unimportant issues can escalate and create real tension between you.

What we are going to concentrate on now are the much more important kinds of arguments.

What are you really angry about?

As we have seen, anger is such a complicated emotion that you yourself might not even know the exact reasons why you are angry. You know the apparent cause – whatever it is that has just happened to make you feel furious – but this isn't always the real reason. If you are aiming to take the heat out of an angry relationship then it is important to be are able to pinpoint what is causing the trouble. Working out what this is can't be done in the middle of a rage and sometimes it is hard to do by yourself. A counsellor is often the best person to help you work through the tangle of emotions that have led to you feeling so angry, and then help you decide what to do about it.

This needs to be done whether you are open about expressing your anger or are busy repressing it. Interestingly, some people who express anger easily are covering up sad or frightened emotions, while their partners who don't rage but seem unhappy or depressed are hiding aggression and fury.

Whatever the apparent reason for your anger with your partner, the causes for feeling so passionate fall into three main areas: things that are happening in your life now that are stressful and difficult; things that happened in the past, perhaps when you were a child, which have not been resolved; and matters directly related to your partner – behaviour or characteristics that you find difficult. Read these sections carefully and see if you can spot any similarities to your own situation.

● **What is happening in your life now.** Frequently your anger reaches a fever pitch when other things are going wrong in your life and you are under strain. A mundane example could be that you have found out that you are overdrawn at the bank or someone has been rude to you. Underneath your anger towards your partner you are really upset over matters that are nothing to do with him or her, but your anger becomes hard to contain because you are upset and disturbed for other reasons.

It becomes particularly hard to handle when the strain you are under is long term: work is going badly, or you are unemployed, or someone you love dearly has died. Other matters that put you under pressure for a considerable period include moving, changing jobs, money worries and problems with your children or older relatives.

Some of these problems cause you to feel unhappy or frightened and if these emotions are hard for you to handle then you are even more likely to fly into a temper. If you are in a situation that you can do nothing to control, such as putting up with an unpleasant boss or suffering long-term unemployment, then you can feel weak and helpless. No one likes feeling this way and it can make you very angry at yourself as well as at the situation.

Men often find it easier to lash out than express feelings of vulnerability or hurt, and it can feel safer to attack the person who must stand by you – your partner – rather than your boss or a government official.

Ask yourself

If you can identify that most of the unpleasant feelings you are now experiencing are to do with matters outside your relationship, then you should ask yourself if you have become too used to taking out frustrations on your partner when they become hard to bear.

Inevitably if you do this your relationship will suffer and things will happen within it to add to your anger. But if you can make yourself explain these other feelings to your partner you might find help rather than strife from your relationship.

If your feelings of anger come about because your partner is aware of your other problems but either appears to be unable to understand them or dismisses them, you also need to talk it through. Usually this means being able to express the deeper emotions behind your anger. For instance, saying that you are 'fed up' because you can't get a job might result in impatience from your partner, who can't understand why you don't put more effort into it. Confessing that you feel afraid that no one will want you and that you fear that you are unemployable (if it that is closer to the truth) will give your partner a clearer idea of what you are feeling. If your partner is behaving in ways that make you feel worse about yourself you must explain what they are. State the facts and what you feel – don't attack and blame your partner for the feelings – and you can then work together on what needs to be changed.

6————————Talking point ————————

Angry moments

Take it in turns to describe to each other your earliest memories of someone being angry with you. How was this shown – by shouting, hitting, weeping, punishing? How did it make you feel – angry too, scared, ill?

Next, take it in turns to describe early memories of witnessing anger between your parents – how did that make you feel? How did they seem to feel? If you don't remember anger being shown in your house, what other feelings were you aware of?

Finally, take it in turns to describe your earliest memories of feeling angry. How did you express it, and what were the consequences?

9

• **What happened to you in the past.** As we have seen, events from your past can sometimes have been so hurtful that you are still carrying around angry feelings about them, letting them spill over into your present relationship. This is the hardest category of anger to identify without a counsellor, but it can help to think back on your family life to see whether there is anything that happened then that still causes you pain.

This was the case with Deidre, who came to counselling when she was on the brink of leaving her husband, who, she felt, gave her so little love that she thought she would be better divorcing him and and taking their daughter with her.

Very early on in counselling Deidre told the counsellor about her angry relationship with her mother. Her mother had been a single parent who had had Deidre at the age of eighteen. Her boyfriend had run off as soon as he had known she was pregnant but she had decided to keep the baby. 'I had you for myself. I needed something for myself,' Deidre's mother often told her, but all Deidre's early memories were of being dumped with her grandmother while her mother went out with other men. Finally Deidre's mother met and married someone else and had another child – a son.

Throughout childhood, Deidre had felt that her brother came first. Her relationship with her mother was always difficult: they quarrelled a lot and Deidre often felt unloved. Her mother's preference for Deidre's brother also soured the relationship between the children; Deidre felt too jealous of the boy to want to get close to him.

The counsellor gave Deidre the task of writing a letter to her mother to tell her everything she had ever felt or suffered. She was not to send the letter but to bring it to the next counselling session and talk it through.

When Deidre arrived for the next session she was elated and excited. She had been sitting down to write the letter when her mother had rung her. During the course of the conversation her mother had said, 'I forgot to send your brother a card on his birthday – isn't that incredible? I can imagine myself forgetting anyone else's birthday, but never his!' Because Deidre had wound herself up to write the letter and knew what she wanted to say, this chance remark had the effect of unlocking her feelings. 'Yes,' she said, 'I've always thought that. You've never loved me as much as him.' From there she went on to tell her mother all the hurts and slights she had felt over the years. Being able to do so made her feel much better. Her mother was taken aback – and defended herself. It gave her the opportunity to talk about her love for Deidre and many other intimate matters.

That was the start of an improvement in Deidre's relationship with her mother and an almost immediate improvement in Deidre's feelings about herself. She gained in confidence, and when that happened she began to get on better with her husband. When the angry feelings about her mother had been dealt with, her relationship with her husband looked better too. She was able to recognise that her husband did love her in a quiet and undemonstrative way, and although there were still matters to sort out she felt optimistic about her marriage.

Angry feelings can also be left over from a previous relationship. Perhaps you were married before or were involved for a long time with someone who behaved in ways that upset you. When your partner does something that echoes this you can become unreasonably angry because it reminds you of the past.

Ask yourself

Are you still experiencing anger or other painful feelings towards someone from your past? If so, then you should ask yourself whether you are interpreting your partner's behaviour in the light of this and perhaps feeling anger that is not really relevant to your current situation.

You could try the task Deidre was given and write to the person concerned about these feelings in the form of a letter which you keep but don't send. In counselling this task is often used to help someone express repressed and angry feelings. Even though the letter is not sent – and even when the person towards whom you feel anger is dead – it helps release the angry feelings that have otherwise been going round and round inside. A direct confrontation such as Deidre had is not always possible or advisable.

It is also worth telling your partner what aspects of his or her behaviour bring these memories back to you. If you say, 'When you do that it reminds me of this particular incident in the past and I find myself getting angry with you,' it is possible for your partner to decide to take this into account and change certain aspects of behaviour.

● **Is it directly related to your partner?** Having examined your feelings, you might be quite clear in your mind that the anger that you feel towards your partner is connected to nothing else but him or her. You are angry quite specifically with your partner.

You could be disagreeing over something major that affects your life together: differences over bringing up the children, one of you wanting to move when the other doesn't, or a major expenditure that only one of you wants to make, and so on. These and other issues can make you very angry and cause rows, but they are all matters that require negotiation. Expressing your angry feelings and listening to your partner's won't get you anywhere unless you are also prepared to work towards a solution that suits you both.

Your anger might be about something that either your partner is doing or has done – an affair for instance. Anger and other emotions on both sides need to be expressed when they concern matters that radically alter your relationship and the way you see each other. Major events of this sort involve a reassessment of your life together and much renegotiation and compromise before you can move forward.

If your anger with your partner is not over any of the major matters mentioned above, but is aroused by many minor points and is a constant feature of your relationship, then it could be the very nature of your partner or the life you have built together that is making you angry.

If you find your partner's personality or opinions and feelings disturbing, you might find yourself embroiled in many rows which have little real cause but which come about through your feelings of general irritation. You might also find yourself becoming unreasonably upset or angry about your partner's personal habits.

Anger of this kind is usually to do with disappointment in your partner or the relationship. A row about who is going to do the washing up can be just that: a practical debate with a short-term goal. But a row about who invented the safety pin, which becomes personal and hurtful, can be a sign that you are unhappy about your partner.

This is sometimes a feature of the 'hangover' period when you have stopped being 'in love' with your partner and have started to see your loved one as real and fallible and no longer perfect. You can't, of course, say 'I'm furious because I wanted you to be my romantic ideal and I wanted to be passionately in love with you forever.' Instead you feel it's legitimate to start a row about leaving toenail clippings in the bath or to criticise your partner for something he or she says or feels. Sometimes these 'hangover' feelings last throughout a relationship and you snipe and quibble at each other over every little matter that arises. Or perhaps the disappointment in your partner occurs some time later in the relationship, when either one of you has changed.

Anger about your partner not being the person you want him or her to be is perhaps the most unfair kind. Everyone is entitled to his or her own feelings and opinions, and to be the person he or she is. You can't change what someone thinks or feels just because you would like to. These angry feelings are *your* problem and you are the only person who can change them – by learning to tolerate who your partner is and changing your expectations of what your partner can be. When you stop having constant rows and start trying to listen to and understand what your partner is like, expressing your disappointment in terms of your own feelings and expectations rather than by blaming your partner for not being different, you have a chance of improving your relationship.

Disappointment over the way your relationship is going can also only be dealt with in this way. Having rows over the little things that annoy you will just increase the bad feelings between you. Stating what you want and need from the relationship and finding out whether you can match this to your partner's wants and needs can provide a solution that works.

! ————————————— *Task* —————————

It gets on my nerves

Make a list of things in your daily life that irritate you and put you in a bad mood. Underneath each make the heading 'It would be better if . . .' and list what someone else could do to remove the irritation. Under this, make the heading 'What I could do . . .' and think of ways you could reduce the irritation for yourself.

Remember, there is *always* something you can do. Solutions include: explaining calmly why you are irritated; removing yourself from the presence of the person who is bothering you; finding practical ways to help the person change his or her behaviour without criticising.

If there is nothing to be done about the situation there is one final thing you can do: say to yourself, 'Nothing can be done to change this so I must stop wasting energy thinking about it'. As the saying goes, 'What you can't cure you must endure.'

!

Ask yourself

Is your anger to do with a matter that can be solved by negotiation? Or is it about things that can't be changed – your partner's personality, for instance? Remember that you have power to make changes in yourself, but you can't force changes on anyone else. If there are things that you don't like about your partner you can teach yourself to come to terms with them. Your partner is the only person who can decide to make changes in his or her behaviour, but it is impossible to change the essential person or the feelings he or she possesses.

How you argue

Whatever your reasons for becoming angry there are helpful and unhelpful ways of dealing with it. Unhelpful ways of arguing – which make matters worse between you and go no way towards solving your problems – are far more numerous than the helpful ways. We look at both ways of arguing here, starting with the unhelpful way.

Personal attack

When you lose your temper you can find yourself saying spiteful, hurtful things to your partner. This is a bad use of anger. You are saying what you hope will cause most pain at that moment, but being personally unpleasant is never helpful.

You might feel momentarily better, especially if you have obviously upset or silenced your partner, but your partner will be feeling angry and resentful, which brings you no closer to a solution. Sometimes you might believe an attack is relevant to the row, or is constructive criticism, but if it judges personality rather than behaviour it is an attack. 'You're so mean' is a personal attack, whereas, 'I feel upset when you don't remember my birthday,' pinpoints an action that can be remedied.

Hurtful words can continue to rankle or distress long after they were said – or even after they have been taken back and apologies have been made. 'Sticks and stones may break my bones but words will never hurt me' is a misleading chant. Words can hurt for years and can break a relationship.

If, however, in the heat of the moment you do say unforgiveable and hurtful things that you don't really mean, you should try to take them back and convince your partner that your anger got the better of you in your desire to hurt. In the same way, you should try to forget unpleasant things your partner says to you. If both of you are genuinely sorry you should make a pact never to use personal attack during an argument.

'———————Talking point ═══════

It's not who wins or loses . . .

When you are angry with each other or disagree passionately over something, it is common to see the situation in terms of a winner and loser – with you, of course, as the one who deserves to win.

But when this happens there is one sure loser – the relationship.

When you set out to win or force your partner round to your point of view the benefits are only short-term. A good result is one that suits you both – and that result is best achieved by negotiation and understanding what it is the other needs and wants. It is this kind of understanding that deepens and enriches a relationship.

Setting out to win at all costs – *especially* if you always succeed – shows a lack of respect, which undermines the foundations of a relationship.

Discuss your feelings about this.

'

• **Insistence on winning.** In the midst of a row you can lose sight of what it was all about and find yourself bent on winning – or beating your opponent. This is usually the time that you stop listening to the other person and concentrate only on your own thoughts and the next attack – you are only hearing your side of the argument.

Some people are in the habit of doing this even when in their heart of hearts they know they are wrong but are nevertheless determined to prove themselves right at all costs. Being able to admit you are wrong is crucial. Until you listen carefully to what your partner is saying, and examine your own motives for saying what you do, you can't be sure that you are right. Insistence on being right stops you reaching a conclusion that will satisfy you both.

• **Moving the goalposts.** This is related to the above: if you are bent on winning at all costs you might change your position half-way through, or deny what you said earlier. Modifying your opinion so as to reach a compromise with your partner is a good thing. Modifying what you say only to remain in the right is another matter all together.

• **You always . . . You never . . . .** This is when a row about something specific enlarges to encompass everything that you feel badly about. You drag up the past and moan about all the habits, irritations and sins, large and small, of your partner.

Couples who row often find most of their rows fall into this pattern.

No matter what issue sparks it off they end up having the same old argument with the same grievances and complaints. Unfortunately nothing is ever resolved in this way. These rows become progressively nastier as time goes on. The only way to vary them is to become more unpleasant in your attack on your partner.

● **Nagging.** We have already covered this elsewhere, but it should be mentioned here. Men nag as much as women, though they may prefer to call it 'reasoning' or 'talking sense into her'.

Naggers take an issue large or small and go on and on about it. Rather than stating their case and point of view emphatically, they are not content to let the subject rest. The result is that people cease to hear what the nagger is saying, and rarely even listen in the first place.

Most naggers believe that they are doing something constructive. However people often resist a nagger by doing precisely the opposite of what is at issue.

● **Hysteria.** Shouting or crying during a row is sometimes inevitable when some of these unhelpful ways of arguing are being used. But once you lose control you will not be able to settle the argument reasonably. Sometimes behaviour like this brings the row to an end, but usually without a solution being reached.

● **Bullying.** Bullying tactics used in an argument might make you temporarily victorious, but they don't change anything underneath. Shouting your partner down, being sarcastic, offensive or hectoring might shut your opponent up, but nothing is solved, only postponed.

● **Blaming.** Blaming your partner for the way you feel inside doesn't help either of you. Saying 'You make me . . .' or 'It's your fault that . . .' puts your partner on the defensive and makes him or her unwilling to listen to your point of view. More importantly it stops you realising that the way you feel is *your* responsibility.

● **Grudge-bearing.** Bringing up any long-gone sins of your partner is also unhelpful. Some people have genuine difficulty in putting past hurts behind them – they never lose clarity, remaining vivid and wounding forever. This kind of person has difficulties because no relationship develops without problems, bad behaviour, or hurtful episodes. Each one will lodge in the mind and heart of an unforgiving person, and if he or she is not going to forget it, then neither will the other partner ever be allowed to.

The important point to bear in mind is that it doesn't help to bring up old grudges time and again. The past can't be changed – it's the present and future you have to work on.

• **Obsessive analysing.** Understanding your own and your partner's feelings and motives is an important part of reaching solutions together. But forcing it on a reluctant partner only creates bad feeling. Being prepared to tell how you feel honestly is your side of the bargain; you can't force your partner to do the same.

One counsellor tells of a husband who insisted on minute examinations of minor aspects of his relationship with his wife. The wife said, 'Sometimes we'd be up until three in the morning going over and over some little thing I'd said, and how it had upset him. He kept asking "But why did you say it? There must be a reason if only a subconscious one." Often I could barely remember the instance let alone the "particular tone of voice" he was complaining about.' The husband eventually came to see that this was a form of emotional bullying, which was getting the opposite result from what he wanted.

• **Physical violence.** It need hardly be said that physical violence doesn't solve any problems in a relationship. It only introduces fear.

Helpful ways of arguing

There are ways that you can continue to express your anger yet get positive results from a confrontation.

• **Keeping the outcome in mind; what do you want to achieve?** The single most important point to keep in mind when you find yourself having an argument is what do you want to achieve?

Do you want to arrive at a practical solution that is agreeable to you both? This is possible if you don't let the anger level rise too high.

Do you want to change the other person's mind? This is less achievable but you can try; remember you are more likely to do so if you remain pleasant and reasonable. After a short time it will be clear whether you will be able to achieve success. If not, stop.

Do you want to get on better or worse with your partner after the argument? If the answer is better, then you have a good reason to steer clear of any unhelpful ways of arguing.

Is there no particular outcome you want? Do you just want to let off steam, complain, relieve your feelings, or make your partner feel as bad as you do? If you are honest enough to recognise that you are picking a fight for the sake of it, with no possible valuable outcome, stop yourself now. Either explain what the real problem is or find another way of relieving your feelings.

• **Taking responsibility for your feelings.** You will be better able to control your temper if you recognise that what you feel is something only you have control over. Your partner might have done something that has upset you, but that does not make him or her responsible for the way you feel about it. Counsellors talk about using 'I messages' rather than 'you messages'.

To take a simple example, your partner might have broken an old plate that was a family heirloom and you are now feeling angry and upset. It is only partly because of your partner's action that you feel upset – it is also because you are sad about the plate and what it meant to you. It is relevant to say, 'I feel upset because you dropped the plate and broke it.' It is blaming to say, 'You made me so upset when you smashed my plate' or worse, 'You're so clumsy, you never take care of things that matter to me – look what you've done now!'

A slightly less clear-cut example could be that your partner turns up hours late for dinner, not having telephoned first. An 'I message' would be, 'I feel so worried when you are late and haven't telephoned. I find myself imagining that you've had an accident or that you might be having an affair. I become so upset and angry that I can't think straight.' A 'you message' might start, 'You're so bloody inconsiderate. It's typical of you just to go off and do what you want without a thought for me. Don't you care whether I'm desperate that you might be run over?', or else, 'Don't start any of your lies with me. I know what you've been up to. I'm not a complete fool, you know.'

A 'you message' is always blaming, and the person who is being blamed will become defensive or aggressive in return. An 'I message' describes the situation in a way that makes the problem mutual: you have certain feelings because of certain actions – what can be done about it? This is very much easier said than done, which is why so few people use this excellent, useful skill. It involves sorting out exactly what it is you do feel, telling your partner truthfully, and doing so without blaming.

It is quite a challenge learning to express what you feel in this way if you have never done so before. The formula has three main parts: state what the specific instance *now* is that has caused the problem, what it makes you feel, and why that is a problem. Where this is something that can be changed you can also ask for help in deciding what to do about it.

A final example: one woman complained in counselling that whenever she came back from a weekend staying with her mother she would find the house a pigsty and the kitchen full of dirty plates. She would immediately launch into a tirade about how useless and selfish her husband was [personal attack] complain about how this always happened [nagging and grudge-bearing] and end up by bursting into tears [hysteria]. Her husband would react by shouting back, telling her she was obsessive about cleanliness and kindly to get off his back and stop spoiling his evening. She would end up cleaning the house till late at night,

...nd furious. As this happened regularly it was clear that her ...ling with her anger had not helped the situation.

... counselling she was able to use the formula to say instead, '... come in and see the place looking a mess [stating the problem], I ... quite exhausted at the prospect of all the work ahead of me after a long drive [what it makes her feel]. That makes me upset and more angry than anything else and because I'm tired I'm likely to go right over the top [why it is a problem].'

Her non-blaming statement achieved her aims. For the first time her husband was able to understand the matter from her point of view; when he had felt under attack he couldn't have cared less how she was feeling. He volunteered to make sure that the place looked OK by giving himself time to clear up before she was due to return. His wife conceded that she was prepared for his work not to be up to her standards so long as the place looked reasonably tidy.

! ═══════════════════ *Task* ═══════════════════

This is what I feel

Explaining what you feel without blaming or criticising the person whose actions have caused your feelings is difficult. Practise using 'I messages' with your partner or a friend when you are in a good mood and willing to have a go. Agree on a time that you are going to do this, and spend half an hour either explaining real feelings, or 'role play' by inventing a situation. You will find this slow to start with, but if you do it regularly you will start to find it easier to express what you want to say quickly.

If you are very angry with your partner and find yourself working up to an argument it can be hard to calm down, use 'I messages' or listen to your partner's point of view. This is a way that can help you.

Before you become embroiled in an argument, write down everything you feel that makes you angry – you can go on for pages if you want to. When you have finished, make a summary of what you have written, no more than one page long. Think about the points you have made and how you could express them without blaming and by using 'I messages'. Talk about them with your partner as soon as you can after this – you will be much calmer if you do. If you have thought through how to explain your feelings you will also find it helpful when you next have a row.

!

- **Being prepared to negotiate.** Expressing your feelings with non-blaming 'I messages' is half the battle. But you must also be prepared to come to some compromise with your partner over certain issues. If you set out to win then your partner obviously has to lose, and when this becomes apparent it is hard for either of you to back down gracefully.

This means listening as carefully to your partner as you want your partner to listen to you. Make a real attempt to understand why your partner feels differently from you on this issue and see if any common ground can be found.

At the end of an argument or disagreement when you think you have found common ground, ask each other whether you feel reasonably happy with what you have decided. If you are dissatisfied with the conclusion, look again together at how you might feel better about it. Can you agree to make any more modifications in your behaviour to bring you closer together?

Effective negotiation also involves understanding your partner's state of mind. Sometimes you might be feeling reasonable, calm, and ready to negotiate, but your partner is more touchy and spoiling for a fight. In these circumstances even a carefully expressed 'I message' can be misinterpreted by your partner as an attack. When feelings are high negotiation will be difficult. It is better to end the argument as quickly as possible and try again another day.

These techniques depend on tolerance, honesty, and a real wish to benefit the relationship − to win the war rather than the battle. If the outcome of a row is that you win at the cost of your partner's wishes or pride then your relationship suffers.

- **Dealing with issues as they arise.** It is easier to use these techniques when you are relatively calm and not in a furious rage. Ensuring that you can cope effectively with matters that make you angry means not waiting for them to come to a head. This involves spotting the warning signs and dealing with them, rather than waiting and having a fight when things have blown out of proportion. It requires developing the habit of talking issues through at an early stage, when you have a niggle of doubt, or are aware of your own feelings of irritation, before matters get out of hand.

Ending the argument

There is little value in an argument that goes on and on. Once you become aware that you are covering the same ground or becoming angrier rather than calmer you have reached the stage when nothing is going to be resolved this time.

Many rows that look as if they are going to become full-scale battles can be shortened dramatically by both of you making a conscious effort to stick to giving 'I messages', listening carefully to each other and negotiating an outcome with which you both can live.

Once it becomes plain that you are not going to be able to reach a successful conclusion and tempers are rising, you should end the argument as soon as possible.

One way is to say, 'We're both getting really upset and angry. This is a problem. Let's leave it now and talk about it again when we're calmer.'

Another way is to agree to disagree. There will always be matters on which you can't reach an agreement, especially when they concern opinions and ideas. Tolerance is important here. You can say, 'I can see how it looks to you. That's not the way I see it, but I respect your view.'

If you find that you have become embroiled in a pointless row that neither of you can win, although both of you are determined to, you must stop as soon as possible. You can try setting yourselves a time limit, 'If we're not getting anywhere in another half an hour, let's stop.'

If you still can't reach agreement then one of you is going to have to let the other have the last word and call a halt that way. Don't consider it a failure if you let your partner have the last word in a row. You can plan to say anything else you want to say when you are both calmer. That way neither of you loses out.

! ═══════════════ *Task* ═══════════════

I don't agree!

Next time you find yourself getting into a disagreement with your partner over something, give yourself a fifteen-minute limit to talk it through. Use a bunch of keys to signify who is talking and who is listening. For five minutes the person holding the keys is allowed to give his or her views on the matter; then the keys are passed to the other while he or she talks for five minutes. Use the last five minutes to try to negotiate an agreement on the matter. If you can't do so, agree to think the matter over and talk about it again another time.

!

Saying sorry

Whatever we are led to believe as children, saying sorry is not a magic charm that wipes out all wrongs. When you have said or done cruel things to your partner saying sorry will not make the hurt go away. You should say sorry when you genuinely regret what you have said or done, but the words alone are not enough. If you are truly sorry you should resolve not to behave in such a way again.

Communication flashpoints

There are as many reasons to make you angry as there are individuals. But some areas of life are more sensitive than others. The next chapter deals with some of the major crisis points that can happen in a relationship.

! ——————————— *Task* ———————————

Peace treaty

If you and your partner are at loggerheads over something, see if you can solve it by drawing up a peace treaty. Both write down the solutions that you want and look at them together. Can you see any changes you can make in your behaviour to bring yourself closer to what the other person wants? Both of you should think of one thing you are prepared to do towards this. Try, step by step, each of you making a concession, to see if you can meet in the middle with a new solution with which you both can live.

!

?_____ Quiz _____

Choosing your words

Look at the following situations and decide which statements or questions are most helpful:

1. You have had a terrible day at work and are feeling depressed and angry. Which question would you prefer?
a) 'Have you had a good day?'
b) 'How was your day?'

2. You have offered to change behaviour that was upsetting your partner. Which comment would make you feel good about it?
a) 'About time too. I can't believe it has taken you so long to understand.'
b) 'Thank you. I feel much better about that now.'

3. You have been turned down for a job you very much wanted. Which response would you prefer?
a) 'Never mind. It's not the end of the world. Cheer up.'
b) 'That must be a disappointment. How do you feel about it?'

4. A book you treasured from your childhood has been given away for jumble. Which response would you prefer?
a) 'It's ridiculous to get upset about such a silly thing!'
b) 'I can see you're upset. What did it mean to you?

5. Someone has been rude to you and you are upset. Which reaction would be most appropriate?
a) 'You don't care what so-and-so thinks!'
b) 'That comment has really got to you, hasn't it?'

6. Something has made you sad. Which reaction would you prefer?
a) 'I know just how you feel. When that happened to me I . . . (etc)'
b) 'Do you want to talk about it?'

7. You have had a gruelling day. Which reaction would you prefer?
a) 'Don't come in here with such a long face. You could try to be pleasant and think about me for a change.'
b) 'Would you like a bit of peace and quiet on your own for a while?'

8. You have started confessing to something about which you are very ashamed. Which response is likely to make you continue talking about it?
a) 'That's terrible! How could you do something like that?'
b) 'I can see this is hard for you to say.'
   Now consider: do *you* say or ask things that are not helpful?

_____ ?

5

CHANGE, PROBLEMS AND CRISES

Even the best matched, happiest couples go through difficult patches in their relationship. Life moves on, things occur that put a strain on you individually or together – and your relationship is usually affected. Whether it suffers or improves because of these happenings depends on many things; what you can be sure of is that it will change.

A problem or crisis can bring matters to a head. Couples who come for counselling usually believe that a particular issue is the 'cause' of trouble between them. Counsellors say that these issues are often symptoms of a more complex, hidden problem to do with the way the couple relates to each other. Sometimes it is only when you look beyond the current symptoms to understand the hidden problem that you can mend your relationship. In this chapter crisis points are looked at individually, in the same way that counsellors will start by exploring the problem that initially brings a couple into counselling. But you should bear in mind that any problem you have needs to be looked at in the context of your entire relationship, and difficulties between you become entrenched if you do not pay attention to the way you are communicating.

CHANGE

Most people are prepared for the fact that major events, such as one of you having an affair, will herald an emotional upheaval and jeopardise or finish a relationship. The main part of this chapter looks at the common crises that can arise in a relationship and various ways of dealing with them positively. But first we look at the impact that change – any change – has on your relationship. Problems and crises naturally force change. But change in itself, even a change for the good, requires adjustment, and this too can be disturbing and uncomfortable.

People are often surprised to find out that stress levels rise even when nice things are happening. A commonly quoted table lists stressful events and gives them points out of 100. This table includes marriage

(50), moving house (50), pregnancy (40) major personal achievement (28), holiday (13), Christmas (12). All of these could happen to a couple who married in July, went away on a honeymoon and then moved into a new house. Within months the wife could be pregnant and the husband be promoted; then Christmas falls at the end of the year. At the finish of an apparently idyllic six months they would find themselves with a score of 193 each. A score of over 150 in a six-month period is excessive and can make you nervous, tense, miserable – even ill. It is worth looking at what it is about change that is so stressful.

Change means upheaval. Whatever is happening is introducing new elements into your life. As you can see from the 'good' changes listed above, it is the changes that are permanent that cause the greatest stress. Holidays and Christmas, which require you to make changes for a short period before getting back to normal, are less stressful than the bigger life changes such as getting married or becoming pregnant.

When something new is happening in your life you have to pause to take stock. If you have been trundling along on automatic, you now have to give some thought to what is happening or about to happen. This demands extra energy on top of your usual requirements. You have to decide in what way you need to behave differently, or how you should cope with differences that have been forced upon you. It produces tension and uncertainty: because these changes are new you can't be sure how you will feel or how well you will cope. Your emotions are affected: they can be up one minute with anticipation and down a moment later because of fear of the unknown, or simply because it is natural for an anti-climax to follow excitement.

These conflicting emotions continue throughout the period of adjustment. Volatile emotions take their toll on your energy and the longer they go on fluctuating the more depleted you will feel. During this period of adjustment your daily routines may be changing and you may need to come to terms with new ways of doing things. The conscious mental effort involved is exhausting.

The sum total of all these new demands is tiredness and sometimes depression – which can be puzzling and upsetting if you feel this way at a time when you think you should be feeling great. After a while everything settles down. The new becomes normal and the extra effort goes out of your daily life. Even so, it is not quite over: now you need a period of recuperation to replenish your energies. If a lot of changes are happening at once, or follow quickly one after the other, it is easy to see that you might not get the time you need to recover properly, and consequently feel frazzled, irritable and physically under par. That means, inevitably, that the people closest to you bear the brunt of what you are feeling.

❛————————Talking point ————————

Grief and mourning

Everyone knows that when someone you love dies you mourn. It is less well understood that you can also mourn and feel grief when major changes happen in your life. You can grieve for the loss of 'your old self' or for a relationship that has finished or for a relationship that has changed so much that it is now different. You can also grieve for places that you have left for good: a family home or the town in which you always lived. You can grieve for lost jobs or for your children's childhood as they grow into adults. Obviously some of these happenings are much less painful and you go through the grieving stages quite quickly, but if you know that this is natural you might be able to better understand what is happening to you. These are the classic stages:

Shock. Obvious symptoms of this stage are not being able to think straight, repeating yourself and forgetting things.

Yearning. You want back what you have lost. You feel anger and sadness and periods of disbelief. You may feel very restless and on edge, full of useless energy.

Depression. As you come to terms with what you have lost you become depressed and apathetic. The energy goes and you can't feel much about anything.

Recovery. You start to adapt to your loss. You stop living in the past and begin to reorganise your life under the new conditions. ❜

The emotional year

This partly explains why annual 'happy' occasions during the year can be disappointing or downright unpleasant. Wedding anniversaries and birthdays, as well as Christmas and holidays, require planning and preparation as well as expense and changes in routine. More significantly, they are occasions when your expectations of pleasure and happiness are very high, activating in you the child for whom these times represented magic and perfection. When reality doesn't match these hopes you react emotionally, not least because there is a whole year to wait before the next occasion. At Christmas, or a family holiday, when a lot of people with high expectations are pitched together in prolonged contact the collective disappointment can inflame any bad feelings that have been smouldering below the surface.

Change in you

Changes in circumstances are easy to pinpoint. But there are also less obvious changes: those inside you as you mature and develop through different life stages. The person that you are is not set in concrete when you reach eighteen, or even twenty-five, thirty, or forty – it never is. Throughout life your needs, outlook, ideals, and sometimes your personality, modify and change. A couple who marry in their twenties and stay together for the next forty or so years will be very different people not simply at the end of it, but at stages along the way. As you change, so you require different things from your relationship. To be able to accommodate these changes in your relationship requires all the elements we mentioned in earlier chapters: humour, respect, generosity, effort, flexibility – and it is a test of how much you like each other as well as the depth of your love. These changes happen whether you hit major snags and crises or not.

Developing at a different pace

Sometimes both of you make developmental changes at roughly the same time. For instance, you both decide you are ready to settle down and therefore want to marry, or both of you feel ready for the responsibilities of parenthood. But quite often you find that one of you is going through a period of change while the other is temporarily stationary. For instance, one of you might be making a breakthrough in your career which involves changes in the way you see yourself and the way others see you: the direction of your life is changing, as are aspects of your personality. Alternatively, you can both be changing in different ways at the same time. For instance, a woman who has spent years as a housewife-mother might go back to work once the children have grown up and have a sense of her life expanding; meanwhile her husband is coping with the fact that he has peaked in his career and is turning back towards the family. Developmental milestones such as the midlife crisis, when you take stock of your life so far and look towards your future in a new way, can affect you both at the same time, or years apart.

All these changes cause your relationship to bend one way and then another in order to accommodate what is happening and the process never leaves it unchanged.

Dealing with change

The changes that make you a different person inside are always difficult to go through. Even when you emerge feeling more mature and happier, the process of getting to that point is not easy. Changes are usually preceded by feelings of frustration and restlessness which spur you into making them. During these times you are focused on your own thoughts and feelings and have less time for your relationship. If you are both struggling with inner changes you might let some of your togetherness lapse and communicate (on the level we talked about in the last chapter) less often or rarely. At a time of inner change it becomes even harder to talk to your partner about what you are experiencing because you haven't yet made sense of it yourself.

If only one of you is going through the process it does not leave the other untouched. At best your partner must be patient and understanding, and also be prepared to make changes although he or she might be content with the way things are. At worst it can cause conflict when your partner feels frightened or angry at the new you which is emerging.

The answer once again comes back to communication. Shutting off from each other makes a needless barrier between you. You don't have to understand your inner turmoil (if that's what it is), you just have to share it. It is perfectly legitimate to say, 'This is what I'm feeling, though I don't know why.' It is also helpful to you to do so. If you don't examine what you are feeling you might project it onto your partner and blame your stirrings of dissatisfaction on someone else, rather than recognising that they come from within you.

Dealing with these changes calls for flexibility – one of the most important elements in an enduring relationship. Give and take is an aspect of this. When a relationship changes because you are going through a difficult period of transition you will need more support than usual from your partner. In a healthy relationship you can take it in turns to see each other through the bad patches. Everyone needs support, even the people who present themselves as ever strong – perhaps those people most of all because they are reluctant to ask for it. In a good relationship you should be able to ask for support from your partner, and give it too.

But, as we saw in earlier chapters, you can be attracted to your partner because he or she has something you lack: the 'marital fit'. If your relationship is too dependent on this fit, it might not have the flexibility to sustain changes.

For this and other reasons some people find *any* change in a relationship unbearable, even if it is for the better. One counsellor cites the case of Fiona and Harry for whom this was so. Fiona initially came for counselling on her own, looking defeated and worn out. Harry, she explained was an overbearing bully. He demanded perfection. When he came home at the end of the day he wanted the house to be immaculate and a meal ready and waiting on the table. He was constantly criticising her. They rowed all the time and Fiona didn't know how long she could carry on. The counsellor said that it was important that Harry should be involved in the counselling, and after four sessions of Fiona coming by herself, Harry reluctantly turned up. Harry's manner bore out everything that Fiona had said. His attitude was irritable and arrogant. His very first statement was, 'I'm coming for Fiona's sake. She's the one with the problem. There's nothing about me that needs to change.'

Gradually a picture of their life together emerged. Fiona had given up work when they planned to start a family, but eventually it had become clear that they were infertile. Fiona had never gone back to work and had settled down as a housewife. But she was a bad manager. Sometimes she would spend all day in bed. She hated shopping and getting it home at all was a triumph. She would leave the shopping bags lined up in their narrow hall for days on end. She had never mastered the art of synchronising a meal so that everything would be ready at the same time.

The counsellor began to see how they grated against each other. Harry would come home from a day's work and immediately trip over the bags of shopping. This would put him in a mood and he would start shouting at Fiona. The meal would be a disaster and they would row again. A sequence of events like this would keep them at each other's throats.

The counsellor felt that it was important for Harry to understand his contribution to the situation. On the question of the shopping bags, she asked him if he could think of another way of handling his irritation rather than shouting. After some thought, he said, 'I could ask her what she wants done with them – if she would like me to put them somewhere.' They went through Fiona's other difficulties, and each time Harry was asked whether there was something he could do to make matters better. He came to understand that in most cases offering to help would make a difference.

The counsellor helped Fiona devise systems that would make things easier. When cooking a meal, for instance, she could prepare the elements separately and then heat them together in the microwave when Harry came home. A number of relatively simple changes on both sides could revolutionise the way they interacted daily and restore harmony to the home.

They came for a number of sessions, reporting back each time on how they had got on. The extraordinary outcome, as far as the counsellor was concerned, was that *Harry* did all the changing – he carried out everything he had agreed to in the counselling room. Fiona, on the other hand, could never manage to make any changes. More curiously, when matters began to improve because of Harry's contribution, she did things that made the situation worse again. She made arrangements to baby-sit for neighbours' children which meant she would not be home when Harry returned from work, and which stopped her from cooking at all. She took on a part-time job and said she could no longer do the shopping.

Tensions in the home rose again. Harry would have another of his rages and she would represent herself as terrified of his bullying demands. The counsellor realised that Fiona couldn't handle Harry's change for the better. She was more comfortable thinking of him as an unreasonable tyrant. When the counsellor tried to help them explore what was happening, Fiona took on new commitments that meant she had no more time for counselling.

Growing apart

Growing apart can happen even when you have tried to hold your relationship together. Sometimes you have developed so differently that you have little left in common. With luck, you and your partner change in complementary fashions, but it is no one's fault if you mature differently, needing and wanting things that are not important to your partner.

Usually, however, you grow apart because life has been too hectic for you to sit down and talk about the changes you have been going through or because you have never learnt good habits of communication.

Counsellors see this most often in marriages that started when the couples were young. Perhaps the couple met as teenagers and started a family soon after. They had to cope with their own growing up alongside the normal difficulties of life and bringing up their family. Often they come for counselling after being married for twenty-five or more years, on the verge of a break-up. The children have left home and, faced with each other alone, they find that they have little in common.

Some couples catch this problem in time, perhaps because a crisis has made them look more carefully at their relationship. With Donald and Loretta it happened when Donald had an affair. As Loretta said, communication between them had all but ceased, 'I would ring up my girlfriends when I wanted to chat about my day – I stopped telling Donald things and having a laugh with him. Our bedtimes got out of synch and sex began to be something we did rather rarely and very hastily. In the end the thought of an evening alone with Donald was more than dull – I thought it was a waste. I only ever looked forward to the times we made up a foursome or had people to dinner.' Until Donald's affair it hadn't occurred to Loretta that there was anything wrong with this, 'I assumed it happened to everyone.'

!
=============== *Task* ===============

I fell in love with you because . . .

If you feel your relationship has gone off course but you are not
sure why, take time to list the reasons you fell in love with your
partner. Be specific. List things that he or she used to do, say or
believe that you found particularly endearing. Than put a cross next
to the ones that have changed. Take time to discuss your lists with
each other. Why have there been changes? What do you both feel
about them?
                                                                !

Taking the relationship for granted

There is something cosy and satisfying about being able to take your
relationship and your partner for granted. In its best sense it means that
you are relaxed and secure in the relationship.

But there is another, less healthy way in which you can take each
other for granted. Because you feel loved and in a relationship that is
built to last you become careless. As in the case of Donald and Loretta,
this can mean ceasing to make the effort to communicate regularly until
you reach a point where you have no idea what is going on in each other's
minds and hearts. When you are going through changes this can lead to
a serious lack of understanding which only grows worse as time goes by.

Taking your partner for granted can also mean that you stop being
even ordinarily considerate. This often happens. You treat each other
rudely and with a lack of respect, increasing the gulf between you. With
hindsight many people whose relationships have reached breaking point
can see that they could have put more effort into making the relationship
work. This involves realising that your partner does not belong to you
and therefore can't be counted on to be around forever if the relationship
between you deteriorates.

Boredom

Some people complain that their relationship has become boring: there
is nothing terribly wrong – no problems or crises – but they have little
pleasure in each other's company and have settled into a dull routine.
People rarely come for counselling at this stage, though many couples
look back at the crisis point and say that it was preceded by a period of
stagnation. Boredom is relevant to a discussion about change. It is
usually the first sign that something needs to change – those stirrings of

restlessness can start to give you the necessary impetus to make changes. You don't have to settle for boredom; some people do, gradually resigning themselves to feeling this way. Neither do you have to end the relationship, though if you make no positive changes the boredom can harden into something more unpleasant and disruptive. What boredom indicates is that your relationship needs attention; it can't just be taken for granted.

Paradoxically, boredom can be a result of change. Most often it is a reaction to the relationship changing from being romantic into something more settled and ordinary. Often there is very little wrong with relationships like this. Some of the best things about a good relationship are, on the face of it, dull. Feeling comfortable with each other, knowing your partner 'inside out', feeling able to 'be yourself', having someone who understands you, and likes you, warts and all – these are not things that make you dizzy with pleasure, but they are important constituents in a strong relationship.

This kind of boredom can happen early in a relationship, or it can take many years to arrive. It is also known as 'the seven-year itch'.

The seven-year itch

The 'itch' classically happens around the seven-year mark, though it can come much earlier or later. The feelings connected with it are experienced by most people in a long-term relationship, but they only sometimes lead to an affair. As one counsellor says, 'I think everyone comes to a point where they feel stuck. But not everyone is tempted into other relationships – except maybe in fantasy – because they have made a commitment. The restlessness, attractions and temptations are there and they have to be acknowledged and talked through. It would be foolish to assume one would go through thirty or forty years of togetherness without periods of dullness or, indeed, meeting other people whom you find attractive or who might have been a suitable partner for you.'

When this occurs during a relationship that is fine apart from run-of-the-mill problems, the cause is often boredom. The relationship has settled down into predictable patterns. The 'itch' is the urge to re-experience excitement, or romance, or perhaps yourself as a sexually attractive being. The trouble with an affair at this time is that it can disrupt a relationship that is just going through a lacklustre stage.

Boredom, however, is not inevitable if you challenge your feelings. You need to look at your restlessness and see it for what it is. For most people who continue to love and value their partners, boredom might only be a sign that they have dropped too radically all the pleasurable elements of courting and intimate communication.

Boredom and hostility

But for some people the end of the romantic stage reveals incompatibility, in which case the onset of boredom is the first sign that the relationship has run its course. Similarly, for reasons of security or convention some people can spend years in a relationship which was never really right for them. Boredom, or the 'itch', can show that they are outgrowing the need for the relationship. This was the situation with Madeleine.

Madeleine was twenty-five and had been married to Patrick for five years. They married at a time when everyone around them seemed to be doing the same. She had thought she was in love with Patrick but it had never been a grand passion – far stronger had been the urge to have a husband and a nice home. They both had good jobs and plenty of money. Neither of them felt ready to start a family. Madeleine said she was quite happy – until she met Nick.

They met at the squash club to which Madeleine belonged. Nick had joined temporarily while he was working in the area. He was charming, clever, outgoing – and an unrepentant rat. He was engaged to a girl back home, was having an affair with a woman at work, and had already slept with two other women at the squash club. Now he was after Madeleine. She did not have an affair with him, but was staggered by the effect he had on her. She said that his attentions, his 'chat', his whole way of being, had touched something in her that had never been touched before.

Madeleine told Patrick how she was feeling. They came for counselling to try to sort things out. Madeleine maintained that what she wanted was for her husband to make her feel the way Nick did. The words she used were, 'I want you to reach me; to touch parts of me you have never touched.' Patrick was distraught and asked Madeleine to tell him what he should do. Her answer was, 'If I have to tell you how to do it then it won't work.' What Nick had given her was a feeling of specialness and excitement, transient things that would not last, but which Patrick had never given her. Madeleine was bored and it became clear that the relationship between her and Patrick was not built on much more than security and convenience.

Nick moved away and Madeleine and Patrick got back to some kind of normality and left counselling. But the counsellor felt unsure about their prospects. Nick coming along had activated the 'itch' but had also drawn attention to an emptiness at the core of the marriage. The counsellor felt that their problems had only been deferred. If something happened to change the fragile balance – Patrick doing less well at work and earning less money, Madeleine's career overtaking his, or if she met someone less obviously a philanderer than Nick – the relationship could break up.

Saying that you find your partner or your relationship boring can sometimes mask a more deep-seated hostility. Some people express anger and resentment by clamming up – and if you don't talk to each other more than is strictly necessary you will undoubtedly be bored by each other's company. Looking at the section on anger in the chapter on Communication can be useful if this is the case. Some people put up with the wrong person in a poor relationship because they prefer it to being alone. The 'itch' at this time is the urge to find a replacement. In these circumstances saying that a relationship is boring is another way of expressing feelings of dislike or disappointment.

Whatever the cause of your boredom – whether you genuinely love your partner and are simply feeling stale, or your relationship has deeper problems – doing nothing about it can make matters worse. Tackling it head on with good communication techniques gives you the chance of improving matters and dealing with problems – and it will certainly dispel the boredom.

Change – how it relates to crises and problems

A crisis or problem in your relationship will cause it to change. But the kinds of changes we have been talking about – developmental changes in the way you think and feel – can also precipitate crises or bring you to a point where you cannot tolerate things you have been prepared to put up with in the past. Although this sounds drastic it can also work as a force for good and move your relationship on to a new, improved phase.

One counsellor tells the story of Jeremy and Beth, for whom individual changes in both of them wrought a radical change in a relationship that had been destructive and unhappy. She says it was one of the most rewarding cases with which she had ever been involved, watching a couple on the verge of breaking up find such value in each other that they fell in love all over again.

Beth had been a shy, inexperienced twenty-six-year-old who saw herself as plain and unmarriageable when she met Jeremy, a suave, handsome man ten years older than herself. He was sophisticated, confident, and, by some miracle (as she saw it) he fell in love with her. She even used the phrase, 'He was my knight in shining armour' – he had come to rescue her from spinsterdom.

Within two years things had gone wrong. Jeremy's job took him travelling and he had his first affair. He was drinking heavily and running up debts. Beth learnt that if he wasn't in by midnight, when he did return he would be so drunk that he would become violent. On these occasions she would drive in her nightclothes to a friend's house for refuge. Over the years matters got worse. His affairs were no secret and they were constantly overdrawn. Partly to help pay their debts and partly to give herself something to do, Beth started to make curtains for extra money.

Ten years after they had married Beth came for counselling. She was now thirty-six and her curtain-making had grown into a successful business. She was very different from the woman who had married Jeremy: she was now confident and she no longer saw a reason to put up with Jeremy's behaviour. Jeremy had changed too. He still drank but was no longer violent. At forty-six he was in the throes of a midlife crisis. He looked and sounded like an old man. Beth wanted to leave him and he had begged her to stay.

For the first ten sessions Beth came to counselling on her own. During that time she realised that she would like to stay with Jeremy, but only if the relationship altered. At this point Jeremy joined them.

It took great effort for them to talk about what had happened in the past. Jeremy recognised how destructively he had behaved but said he had not fully realised before how it had affected Beth. They had lost the habit of talking to each other, and needed to relearn it. Jeremy would say to the counsellor about Beth, 'I love her'; the counsellor would ask him to tell Beth himself. Beth, too, had to explain to Jeremy how she felt, not direct her comments through the counsellor. The counsellor never criticised. She pointed out that behaviour was not good or bad; it was helpful or unhelpful. If you knew the consequences you had the choice – to behave as you always had or to do it differently.

They took new ways of communicating back home. In the past Jeremy, ignoring Beth, would walk into the house, collapse in front of the TV and doze all evening. Now he would greet her and they would kiss. They would spend the evening talking together, about ordinary matters as well as what they were going through.

The counsellor says that at every session she could see the love growing between Beth and Jeremy, their intimacy deepening through their new ways of communicating with each other. Jeremy gave up drinking and the counsellor asked him how they could know that it would last. What would stop him drinking? Jeremy said, 'I know now what I stand to lose. Beth matters to me too much. If I drink she might go.' The counsellor says she will always remember the starry-eyed look that Beth gave Jeremy at that moment.

As their relationship improved, so Jeremy stopped acting like an old man. He made an effort with his appearance and his confidence returned. For the first time the relationship achieved a balance. Initially, Jeremy had been the strong one, 'in charge' of the relationship, then it had swung the other way. Now they could see that they needed each other: they had an equal investment in the relationship and were also gaining real pleasure from each other. By the end of the counselling Beth and Jeremy were excited and happy about the direction their relationship had taken. The counsellor says, 'It was like first love – but much more solid.'

?————————Quiz————————

I've changed, you've changed

If you have been together for some years it is natural for some of your
views on certain matters to have changed. This quick quiz looks at some
of the main areas that could be affected. Look at the questions and tick
the answer nearest to how you felt when you first met, and then answer
them again as you feel now. Discuss together any points on which you
do feel differently nowadays.

	Her		Him	
	then	now	then	now

Children
Want them now/have them
Want them some time
Never want them

Money
Not important to me
Quite important to me
Very important to me

Work
Don't want to work
Just do it for the money
I'm ambitious and want to get on

Relationship
The two most important elements are:
Sex
Romance
Companionship
Security

Home is . . .
A haven of rest
The centre of family life
A base: life happens elsewhere

What I want most from life
To enjoy myself
To do something really worthwhile
A quiet life without problems

————————————————————————————————?

PROBLEMS

Daily life brings problems. Some of them can be sorted out. Others are intractable and last for years, becoming a feature of daily life. These are not crises: either the matter is too small to be so classified, or too enduring. A crisis is a major happening and although the after-effects can be long-term, the event itself rarely is.

The wear and tear of ordinary problems take their toll as much as any crisis. They can come between you if you let them – but they can also unite you more closely than happy events. Weathering bad times together, sharing your thoughts and feelings on them, working through solutions – even learning to endure what can't be improved – all add depth and commitment to a relationship. Every time you face a problem together and come through it your relationship is strengthened. You have shown yourselves that you can survive difficulties, and that gives you courage to deal with others that might come along.

Facing problems

To survive these difficulties, the problems must be faced. Ignoring problems in the sense of not making real efforts to deal with them together – or arguing about them rather than trying to find solutions – is common.

Fear lies behind most reasons for not dealing effectively with problems. Fear of the changes you might have to make in your life and your relationship in order to do something about your difficulties. Fear of the problem itself – hoping that if you carry on as if it didn't exist it might go away of its own accord. Fear of your own and your partner's unhappy feelings, which you believe will be unbearable if aired. Fear of your own ability to cope, making you put off the moment of having to try. Fear of breaking up because the problem has been brought out into the open.

Sometimes a basically sound relationship breaks up because the couple has never appreciated that ups and downs are inevitable. The difficulties and pain that problems bring are seen to be a sign that the relationship itself is at fault.

Your problems are unique to your situation. It is not useful to list all possible potential problems and all possible solutions. But in a special category are money problems and problems with your children, which are common to many people. These problems fill books on their own, but it is useful to briefly look at some of the points they raise.

● **Money problems.** These can place an intolerable burden on you. The issue becomes survival, so worrying about whether your relationship is working or not might seem a luxury you are not able to afford. Two anxious or frightened people locked together in a difficult situation are likely to take it out on each other, even when love and friendship have been there in quantity.

If your problem is too little money the daily pressures sap your energies, making you feel trapped and dependent on each other. It is most important to be able to talk about it and decide together how you can tackle the problems it causes.

Many couples come to Relate because they are fighting about money – not just those who are on the breadline. Some money problems turn out to be simply a matter of budgeting. If neither of you is good at it, sitting down with a sensible outsider – not necessarily a counsellor – and working out what needs to be done can solve this. Listing what you spend is a practical way of working out your own budget. One counsellor recalls a couple who rowed continuously about the fact that the young wife could never make her housekeeping money last the week. She suggested that the wife wrote down everything she spent in the course of a week. In their case the wife was careful and thrifty, and her husband was able to see for himself that everything cost more than he had supposed. They allocated more of their budget to housekeeping, and the rows stopped.

But friction over money sometimes reveals a difference in priorities. One of you complains about what the other spends money on because you feel it is needed elsewhere. Very different attitudes to spending, saving, accounting and budgeting are a real problem because money affects every aspect of ordinary life. Compromises need to be reached on the various aspects of money management if you are not going to be fighting all the time.

Occasionally, rowing about money masks another problem altogether. One couple came for counselling because they had financial problems which, they said, were undermining their relationship. At one point the counsellor went through all their income and expenditure with them and discovered £65 a week unaccounted for. It turned out that this was what the man spent every week on alcohol. It was not a secret from his wife, but until they came for counselling over their financial differences they had colluded to ignore the fact that drink was the problem.

● **Children.** Differences of opinion over the way you bring up your children are rooted in your own past. Your childhood, good or bad, affects the way you want to bring up your own children, whether you want to do it the same way your parents did or whether you strive to be different. Sometimes you won't know until the children arrive how strongly you feel about this.

This is one of the prime issues for which careful negotiation is necessary. If you don't reach a compromise – or a series of compromises as the children grow up – it will be a perpetual battlefield. That's not good for your relationship, and it is certainly not good for the children. Bringing communication skills to bear on the problem will help you to resolve it and be an excellent example to your children.

Children coming along can also activate feelings of jealousy. You are no longer the only important people in each other's lives – you are parents too, and either one of you might feel jealous of your partner's deep and loving attachment to the children. Many people find this jealousy difficult to express because they are ashamed of it or because they haven't fully recognised it for what it is. If it is ignored the result is often displaced anger, when you quarrel about other, minor matters, or perhaps take it out on the children with excessive discipline or by withdrawing love. Left undealt with for years it can take you far away from your partner emotionally. Many couples come for counselling when the children have almost literally come between them – they relate to their children but rarely to each other – or when one or other of the parents is the go-between for the whole family. A mother might find herself liaising between the children and the father, who never directly makes his own relationship with them.

In a healthily operating family each member makes a unique relationship with every other member. It is a challenging balancing act which requires effort when your life is very busy. Couples often need reminding that they are still entitled to privacy and time to keep their own relationship alive amidst their commitments to their children. Counsellors urge them to make time alone regularly – however difficult – so that they can do this. They need to be reassured that this time 'taken' from the children benefits the whole family: a loving relationship between you gives your children the best example to follow, and is one of the most important elements in helping them form good relationships when they are grown-up.

Similarly, if each of you is able to make some time for your children individually, the family unit is strengthened. Communication skills are equally relevant here: children need to be listened to and respected as well as talked at. They need you to be a human being, warts and all, not a god-like figure who is never wrong. Children who are respected and whose individuality is understood and tolerated are more likely to be respectful and tolerant in their turn.

The best communication skills in the world won't ensure an unruffled family life. There will always be practical problems and ups and downs in family life: problems with schools, allocation of time, adolescents testing themselves against you, as well as the inevitable family arguments. But your best efforts won't go unrewarded if tackled with good communication skills: the problems will resolve themselves and the relationships you make will last after your children leave home because they are based on respect and friendship as well as love.

Life as a family will always have its problems, but sometimes counsellors see couples who are having difficulties and blame them all on one of the children.

As one counsellor says, 'It's all they want to talk about. It gradually becomes clear how vitally this child operates in the marriage as the focus of all the bad feelings that they can't express to each other. Often I find that their sex life has broken down – and it's the child's fault again: "I'm so worried, or so tired because of the child that I really don't feel I want to make love"!'

Usually the child *is* very difficult, but this is fostered by the attitudes of the parents. They are constantly irritated or angry at the child, or move between being over strict and then compensating by being too indulgent until something makes them snap again.

Susan and Howard blamed all their problems on Marty, their toddler, a lively, difficult child. Until Marty had become a problem everything in their lives had followed a pre-set pattern. They had become engaged, saved up for a deposit on a house while Susan accumulated her 'bottom drawer' and only then had they married. Susan's pregnancy went to plan, as did the birth. They strove to do everything 'by the book'. The two-year-old was the one thing they couldn't control.

Through counselling it emerged that Susan found it difficult coping with mess of any sort: her own mess, her husband's mess, messy emotions – anything that raised feelings of not being in control. Three years into it, her marriage no longer seemed picture-book. Her own parents had had an unhappy marriage and unless hers was perfect she feared that it too would go out of control. She had been unable to face these fears, never mind share them with Howard, so they began to centre on that least controllable of beings – the toddler.

Susan and Howard came when their problem was still in its early stages, and the insights they gained meant that they stopped blaming Marty and started to look at themselves and their relationship realistically. Many people, of course, don't come for counselling at this stage, so that a problem that starts with the child becomes entrenched, the child becomes even more difficult, and they fail to see their contribution to the situation.

● **Sex.** Problems with your sex life are usually related to other problems between you, but your dissatisfaction can become focused on the sexual element. The impact of this, and what to do about it, are dealt with fully in the chapter on Sex.

CRISIS

A crisis is different from the slow-growing doubts wrought by changes and the continuing pressure of long-term problems. Its effects are dramatic; the upheaval and emotional consequences are violent. Perhaps one of you has an affair, or there is an unplanned pregnancy. It could be that one of you has a job offer in another part of the country, or is made redundant, or wants a change of life-direction that affects the other.

No crisis need mean the end of the relationship. Even an affair, which is in a special category, doesn't have to be the cause of a final split. In each case it depends how deeply you feel about the issue and each other and how you deal with it.

Whatever the crisis, you must deal with it together. This can be hard to put into practice, particularly as you will both be under strain and not at your best.

At times like this you tend to fight rather than reason. Sometimes it is only when the worst is over that you can begin to look at the causes and the effects.

A crisis can come out of the blue or be symptomatic of other problems. An infidelity might be unimportant or a drunken fling. But it could also be the sign of restlessness or a strong desire to leave the relationship – a feeling that was already present. The need to change the nature of the relationship can mean that one partner engineers a crisis. Even when a crisis occurs in a previously contented relationship – a pregnancy that is a genuine mistake, or a redundancy, it can be the catalyst that makes you look more closely at your partner and your relationship.

Inevitably staying together after a crisis involves compromise and often a radically changed relationship. You can't wish the affair away, or magic a new job, or change fundamental feelings about wanting children or needing independence.

Some of the common crises are now detailed individually. Yours might not be here, but the way to deal with it is always the same: honest and prolonged communication. A strong, good relationship can survive almost any crisis if the will is there.

YOUR FIRST CHILD

If you haven't yet had a baby, you might be surprised to see this included in a section on crises. But the birth of your first child is the single most life-changing event that can happen to you, particularly if you are a woman, but also if you are a man. As we have seen, the greater, more long-term changes you have to make the greater the upheaval in your life, and this affects you physically and emotionally. Even couples who adore their babies, for whom pregnancy and birth go smoothly and whose baby is as good as gold, will have to contend with the changes this makes to their lifestyles and their feelings about themselves, each other, their relationship and the future. It is understandable that many women go through a period of depression after the birth, and even those who don't will occasionally feel under pressure and swamped. New fathers will also find the strain difficult at times and, if this is ignored, the relationship between the couple can hit a rocky patch. People without children might think all this is unnecessarily gloomy. Isn't having a baby the most wonderful thing that can happen to a couple? Don't people have children to bring them together, not to cause problems between them?

There is truth in this, but not the whole truth. Knowing the down side of having a baby won't take away one bit of the pleasure, excitement and love you will feel. But *not* knowing that having a baby means difficulties and causes you to feel all sorts of conflicting emotions brings its own troubles. If new parents find themselves suffering symptoms of stress when they are expecting to feel happy it can be very disturbing. A couple can feel guilty, abnormal, or not fit to be parents when alongside the love they feel a degree of depression, apprehension, misery or anger. Because of the guilt and the belief that this shouldn't be happening they can find it difficult to talk to anyone – even to each other – about what they are going through. And it is when these feelings are unacknowledged that problems start. You can withdraw into yourself or turn against your partner at precisely the time you need each other's strength.

Before we look at ways to deal with this period of adjustment, we need to look more closely at why it can be a difficult time.

Your expectations

Whatever your reasons for having a baby: practical (you are married and you have always believed that marriage is about having children); emotional (one of you is feeling broody); or accidental (it just happened); the stage of planning for a baby can be one of exceptionally loving closeness for a couple.

It is a time of sky-high expectations. An unborn child is an ideal child. Becoming parents is a chance to right all the wrongs of the past – be better parents than yours were – while incorporating all the good things you remember from childhood.

You might have fears about the health of your unborn baby, but no one envisages a difficult child or imagines themselves not having the qualities to be good parents. Even if people tell you of their own difficulties, or you see them struggling with parenthood, the tendency is to think that it won't happen to you, or you will manage better.

Your first baby is a unique experience in your life; no one can prepare you for it. You can't even imagine what it is like, let alone equate it to your experience with other people's children. No two people react in the same way to parenthood. Your baby is unique, and the mere fact of becoming a parent changes you. You can only guess at how it will affect you.

Many people, at the moment their child is born, feel everything they had hoped: they feel excited and elated and unusually clever. Other people, perhaps women who have had difficult births, may feel unhappy and angry – and sometimes frightened because they don't feel an immediate mother love. Whichever way the birth of your baby affects you, it also has a much deeper impact. Having a baby is irreversible: you can divorce your partner, sell your house, leave your job or the country – but you will now be a parent for life. For women this truth has an even greater significance as it is still the case that in the majority of broken relationships it is the woman who will keep the children.

Changes

The baby makes changes in all areas of your life. In practical terms it has a radical impact on your daily routine and on most of the ways in which you operate as a couple. The emotional changes are more far-reaching, because of the difference in the way you come to see yourselves and each other.

Practical changes

Everyone knows that a new baby is going to turn their lives upside down at the beginning. But some people are unprepared for the tiredness that they feel. The mother has undergone the equivalent of a major operation, yet instead of spending her time resting and being looked after she is on twenty-four-hour duty, only snatching odd hours of sleep. The father's sleeping pattern is similarly disrupted, and more of the chores can fall to him.

Even when this most tiring phase has passed, life is very different. Most women give up work for the foreseeable future, and even those who go straight back after maternity leave find that life has changed: now they have to deal with child-care arrangements on top of everything else.

Whether the mother goes back to work or not, a baby coming along means much less money. The loss of the wife's income is balanced by the working mother having to fork out for child-care, and the baby adds

expenses of its own (the more money you have the more you c.
spend on the baby) so it is a time of financial pressure.

Less money is accompanied by less time. A baby takes a l
looking after, even the one who sleeps most of the time. One counsellor
tells of a mother who had many plans for what she would do in between
the times when the baby was asleep but found that she could never get
round to any of them. She kept a diary for two or three days, writing
down exactly what she did and when, and was relieved to see in black
and white how busy she had been kept; some women do the same so
that they can show their husbands who can't believe a baby takes up so
much time.

There is also less time for you as a couple. Simply doing things and
getting out of the house together become major tactical operations – even
if you have enough energy or money to do so!

The impact of these physical and practical changes – the tiredness,
the extra work, the changes in routine, the disorganising of pleasant
times spent together – result in further emotional ups and downs. These
are happening alongside emotional changes of a much deeper nature as
you come to terms with becoming a parent.

!———————————— *Task* ————————————

The reality

If your baby has already been born, list the changes that the baby
has meant to your life under these headings:

Work
Energy/tiredness
Social life
Sex life
Time together
Money
Feelings about myself
Other

Put a tick by the changes you expected and a cross by the
ones that took you by surprise. Look at your lists together and
discuss how they make you feel.

If you have not yet had a baby, write lists under these
headings of the way you imagine things will be. Put them away and
look at them again when the baby is a few months old. Had you
anticipated the changes? Are there any surprising ones?

!

Becoming parents

Having a baby automatically turns you into a parent, but the realisation of what this means in your life often dawns more slowly. This is when many people first feel truly adult. The responsibility for another human being who depends totally on you means that you have to say goodbye to some of the more carefree aspects of your life. This responsibility affects men and women in different ways, so we will look at these separately before examining how they affect you as a couple.

● **Becoming a mother.** The main responsibility for the day-to-day care of the baby is nearly always the mother's. Women are expected to know how to look after babies. In practice, most women have had very little experience of babies before they have their own. In the past, when families were larger and people lived in family communities, most girls had lots of experience of looking after children with their younger brothers and sisters and other members of the family. By the time their own children were born they had a good idea of what to do. Nowadays, when you might have to be taught even how to hold your baby, as well as the practical details of feeding, changing and bathing, it can be a shock that it doesn't come naturally. If you find the mechanics of the care of a small baby difficult, and perhaps also feel as much misery as mother love, you might worry that you haven't got what it takes to be a mother.

Nevertheless, you have to learn to think of yourself as a mother. This process can be slower than you imagine. Feeling like a mother deep down – rather than simply acting like one – involves changing the way you see yourself. This can take months to happen – it certainly isn't automatic with the birth of your child – and getting used to the fact can be disturbing. Some women make the psychological changeover quite quickly, but for others it can take much longer and be one of the causes of postnatal depression.

It is disturbing because so much has changed forever in your life, and in many ways you are going to be a different person. Feeling so different that you are no longer sure you really know yourself is uncomfortable. Until you have come to terms with the changes you are likely to feel churned up and emotionally touchy, and this is happening when you are physically low and emotionally vulnerable.

A baby is part of you: physically while you are pregnant, and then as a constant presence for months afterwards. You have to become used to thinking about the baby's needs at all times, when previously your own needs were your main concern, and other people's needs only mattered intermittently.

Women who recognise that in many ways they have changed forever make this transition more quickly and with less anxiety. It is harder if you think that what is happening to you is temporary, and that you will get back to 'normal'. If by this you mean feeling, looking and behaving exactly as you did before you became a mother, you will be disappointed. Life will settle into a normal pattern, but it will be different and in many ways better.

It is also easier to adjust if you do not set yourself too high standards of mothering. Accepting that mothers learn by mistakes and can't be perfect allows you to feel relaxed about being a mother sooner. This can be difficult if you are used to being efficient and in control. Babies are not subject to reason in the same way as you, your work, or your partner are. Letting go and being flexible helps the whole process of adaptation.

?_____Quiz_____

A boy for you, a girl for me

If you don't have children, play the following game. Answer the questions pretending that *you are your partner*.

1. The number of children I want is . . . (you can put 0 if that's what you think)
2. The number of boys I want is . . .
3. The number of girls I want is . . .
4. I want:
a) a boy first; b) a girl first; c) doesn't matter;
5. I would like my first baby to be born before (date) . . . .
6. My first choice for a girl's name is . . . .
7. My first choice for a boy's name is . . . .
8. I think:
a) the mother should carry on working; b) the mother should not work for a time; c) the mother should not work at all;
9. I think:
a) care of the baby should be shared; b) the mother should do most of the caring; c) the mother should do all the caring;
10. The father should: (tick as many as you think)
a) change nappies; b) bath baby; c) prepare feeds; d) get up in the night for baby; e) take baby to park; f) put baby to bed; g) support mother and baby financially

Now compare answers. Did you get them right?

_____?

● **Becoming a father.** The upheavals in the father's life are not so radical as in the mother's. If he works there is still his job to go to, and most of the care of the baby is carried out by his partner.

But emotionally the changes affect him just as deeply. The burden of financial responsibility for the mother and the baby can seem heavy and frightening. Your job and earning power matter more than ever before. If, previously, your partner worked, your wages have had to cover only your share of the outgoings; now two people are dependent on you. The changes this must mean in your attitude to work can be sobering: having a baby makes a career and position in the world seem vital. You can no longer fantasise about telling the boss where to put his job when it is getting you down, or think about throwing it all over to go round the world.

While having a baby can make a man feel proud and joyous, becoming a father can also appear to bring problems without the same rewards as mothering. What does a father do in the months after the baby is born? You can feel close and necessary to your wife as she gives birth, but after that your role is less tangible. Mother and baby are becoming a unit, and your efforts to help can seem clumsy and useless. If your own father was emotionally distant or absent altogether you might have little idea what a father can do to become close to his children, however much you might want to.

Your changing relationship

Your different ways of struggling to come to terms with becoming a parent and the changes in your life and routine are bound to affect your relationship.

A baby changes the balance of a relationship in a number of ways. Firstly, it can tie you together even more securely than marriage vows. The majority of people feel even more committed to making their relationship work once they have children. The bond between you, initially composed of love, now has a stronger element of duty. This can be unnerving in itself if, until now, feelings of responsibility and duty have hardly figured in your life.

It is also a time when a woman becomes most aware of how much she needs her partner: having a baby means that you now need your relationship with your partner to continue more than ever. In practical terms you might have given up work and now be relying solely on his income. Even if this delights him, you lose the freedom to spend as the fancy takes you. If you have been used to arranging your life as you please, you might also feel temporarily trapped in the home by the baby. This makes you need your partner's support more than ever – to feel reassured that he still loves you. You might find this new dependency frightening, which can affect the ease with which you relate to him.

Men too can find that they need more emotional reassurance from their partners, now that all the attention that used to be focused on them is shared with the baby. In fact, the arrival of a baby often brings out the need in both of you to be shown that you are loved and cared for, at a time when circumstances make it difficult for you to give each other the time to do so.

All this is complicated by the fact that just as you have to learn to see yourself as a mother or a father, so you have to accept that your partner is no longer 'just' your partner but a parent too.

As we have seen in earlier chapters, becoming a parent can make you behave very differently, as you 'act out' your ideas of how a parent should behave, based on your experiences within your own family. Things about your partner that used to enchant you might now irritate: for instance, the woman might want the man to behave more like a grown-up, when previously she enjoyed his boyishness, or the man might start feeling angry that his partner is not a better cook and housekeeper (as he believes mothers should be) although it never bothered him before. On the other hand, you might mind the changes that your partner is making as he or she grows into the new parental role – when you would rather that he or she remained the same person with whom you fell in love. And if part of you believes that it is inappropriate to act lovingly towards each other once you become parents, you can start to grow apart gradually without you realising it.

Mixed feelings

All this means that the birth of a baby can arouse very powerful mixed feelings in you. There are times when you are overwhelmed by love, happiness, pleasure and excitement and other times when you feel the reverse: anger, misery, depression and anticlimax. It can be frightening when some of these feelings are focused on the baby. At an emotionally turbulent time it is understandable that the baby can sometimes arouse negative feelings in you, but it is shocking if you have not expected this to happen. If you are feeling very tired and low and the baby keeps on crying or is sick when you have just cleaned up you can instinctively feel angry, even though you are well aware that it is not the baby's fault. As one mother says, 'I had always thought of myself as a gentle, kind person but I sometimes felt such boiling feelings of rage and even hate for the baby I loved so much that I feared I might do him harm. Of course I never did, but for the first time I was able to understand why some people batter their babies.'

Such intense feelings are normal, and they do pass. But parents who have experienced them feel guilty and upset, and sometimes too ashamed to tell anyone how they feel.

These mixed feelings also spill over into your relationship. Sometimes you can feel that along with your gains you have also lost something. If your relationship has become more stressed, feelings of intimacy might temporarily be absent, just when you need more reassurance.

Because of this, either of you might experience jealousy. The mother might feel jealous because when she was pregnant she was the centre of attention, which has now moved onto the baby. She might feel that her partner almost ignores her when he comes in and makes straight for the cot. She can feel that she is only regarded in so far as she is a good mother to the child.

The new father might also be jealous of his partner's attachment to the baby and feel pushed out by the child – or jealous because the baby is bonding more closely to the mother than to him. Either way, he feels excluded from a deeply intimate and physical relationship. It is at this time that women who have good relationships with their families also tend to turn back to their mothers for support, something else that can make their partners feel redundant and pushed out.

Perhaps it is for these reasons that sometimes the man will embark on an affair during this period, which deals the relationship a blow at an unusually sensitive moment. It can be hard for the new mother to understand the depths of her partner's conflicting feelings about parenthood and the changes the child has made in his life when she is struggling with so much herself. It can seem like the ultimate betrayal. Counselling can put the affair into perspective and help the couple deal with all the emotions surrounding the birth of the baby, as well as the affair itself.

! ─────────────── *Task* ───────────────

The good and the bad

If your baby has already been born, make two lists under the headings:

The best things about my baby

The worst things about my baby

Don't be ashamed to write your true feelings under the second heading – everyone has something to say here. Discuss your lists together.

!

Sex

Your sex life always changes at this time. Changes can start during the latter stages of pregnancy when finding comfortable positions for lovemaking is harder. Some couples stop making love even earlier than this, either for medical reasons or because they are worrying unnecessarily that sex will harm the unborn child. After the birth it takes time for the woman to be ready for sex for various reasons. This can cause concern: if sex has always been the main way you have expressed your love for each other, you might now feel isolated. The man can feel that his partner's unreadiness for sex proves that he has been pushed out by the baby, and the woman can miss the loving, physical attention of her partner if he feels that cuddling, kissing and intimate chat have to be avoided as well as sex.

● **The physical problems.** Giving birth leaves a woman stretched, tender and with perhaps stiches or tears to heal, so that penetration is painful or at least uncomfortable. She may continue to bleed for a few weeks, and quite heavily at the beginning.

It used to be said that you couldn't make love for six weeks after the baby was born, but now doctors are more flexible. Usually you are asked to wait until after your postnatal check-up before resuming.

Until healing is complete, a woman is likely to be sore, and the skin in the genital area can be tight and prickly. As stitches and tears heal they form temporary scar tissue, which may feel tight. Even when everything has healed, there often remains a tender area at the base of the vagina near the anus, which may take longer to feel normal.

You may find that discomfort during intercourse continues until you are fully recovered, which can take some time even if you have healed well. Normal sex can be uncomfortable for as much as six months, but if pain or discomfort continue you should consult your doctor.

Tiredness can also affect the level of desire in both of you. In some cases hormones are to blame for a woman temporarily losing desire. Prolactin – the hormone that controls breast-feeding – can inhibit sexual response. Sometimes doctors will prescribe artificial hormones for a time to right the balance.

● **The emotional problems.** It is more common than is usually realised for women to go off sex for a while after the birth of a baby, even when there is no physical problem. This usually rights itself within months, but for a few women it can go on for years. Women to whom this happens report that lust just disappears, and that they don't like the idea of sex, even when they previously enjoyed it.

There are good biological reasons for this: it guards the woman from becoming pregnant again too quickly. It also means that she is more focused on forming the important bond with her baby.

But there are also psychological factors that can turn a woman off sex. Some women feel unattractive after the baby is born. If you are overweight, tired and harassed, you can find it difficult to respond sexually. Once you regain confidence in yourself your sexual feelings usually return. In a few cases, women who have had difficult births continue to blame their partners for what they have suffered, and these hostile feelings also inhibit desire. Similarly, if you feel that all the responsibility of the baby is yours, and your partner is not prepared to help, you may find that anger saps your sexual feelings.

Some women are frightened when they find they have lost desire, and their men feel rejected and confused. It helps to know that desire does return, especially if the relationship is otherwise good.

Sometimes it is the man who finds that his sexual feelings change. A minority go off the idea of sex after watching the birth. A few become temporarily impotent after this experience.

Even men who are quite able to make love sometimes find that they look at their wives' bodies in a different way, and it takes them time to recapture the image of their wives as sexual beings.

A man's sexual feelings can also be affected by jealousy, which can sometimes be sparked off by watching his partner breast-feed. A jealous man may express his hostility by not appearing to be interested in sex, or by wanting it at moments when the baby needs attention.

Some men want sex with their partners very much but are reluctant to resume lovemaking in case they hurt their partners. They worry that they may cause them to tear, or suffer in some way.

Either of you can find that your feelings about the appropriateness of lovemaking change when you become parents. Perhaps because of ideas developed during your childhood you might feel that sex is all right for people before they have children but not after. Your feelings about your partner can become confused by these ideas. A man might find he can't see the mother of his child as a 'sex object'; making love to a 'mother' seems wrong. A woman can feel the same about sex with a man who is now also 'father'.

Re-establishing your sex life

There are also practical problems when it comes to starting up your sex life again. After a gap, spontaneity is lost, and a decision has to be made to start again. This can be difficult if you are not in the habit of talking about sex.

Both of you will feel much more tired than usual. For a few weeks a young baby wakes regularly throughout the night. This is physically draining – and while you are listening out for the baby it is difficult to relax during sex.

It is important to talk about the loss of sexual desire or other sexual issues. The chapter on Communication will help here.

If one or both of you can't face sex at the moment, it doesn't mean that your physical relationship must cease. Loving, physical closeness that includes affectionate touching, cuddling, and kissing is reassuring at this time. Even if penetration is impossible or difficult, you can still have an active sex life if both of you want it. There are many other ways of giving each other sexual satisfaction, and this is an ideal opportunity to experiment with other forms of lovemaking. If you continue to touch and receive erotic pleasure from each other then resuming a full sexual relationship can be allowed to happen in its own time, quite naturally. For further ideas, look at the chapter on Sex.

Adjusting happily to parenthood

To come through this period well it is important to keep your relationship close. If you have fears, problems, or hostile feelings, you may be inclined to keep them to yourself. But talking is as important now as ever. The chapter on Communication can help you with expressing and dealing with negative feelings. If either of you feel less than thrilled by the new baby it also helps to say so – and to know that this too is normal and usually passes.

Before you start . . .

If you are reading this before becoming pregnant it gives you an ideal opportunity to think and talk about the points that have been raised. Talking about your expectations of parenthood and your attitude to it won't mean that you will have no adjustment difficulties, but it will help keep the lines of communication open. Some people never think or talk about the reality of a baby before it arrives and this can make it harder for them to deal with problems that then arise.

Talk about the impact it will make on your lives in terms of practical changes and financial implications. Make the decision when to have the baby together. During counselling it often emerges that most first children are conceived because the mother wants a child and the father simply goes along with this. If you are both fully involved with the decision you can see the importance of following it through by both of you sharing in the care of the child when it is born.

Becoming a family

When your child arrives you have become a family. There is now a third person, someone to love and with whom you both must relate.

Couples who recognise that the father is very important in the process of creating a family usually make a good adjustment to the birth of a baby. If both of you are involved in the care as well as in the responsibilities you will also grow closer together.

In many ways it is harder for the father to make a real contribution. Preconceived ideas about masculine roles are often at odds with being a good father. Fathers need to be gentle and in touch with their softer, loving, emotional side, and if either of you feel this is unmanly it can be difficult to do.

For practical reasons it can be hard too. The father might be at work and have very little time with the baby. Some women are also very protective of their roles as mothers. They say they want their partners to help but then make them feel inadequate and inept when they try. Making time for the father to be at home with the baby after birth helps. Some employers allow a day or two of paternity leave, and it might be possible to take some of your holiday at this time. Weekends or other time off can be used to get to know the baby better and the mother should be prepared to stand back and allow her partner to develop his own relationship and ways of doing things with the baby. Getting to love and be loved by the baby – bonding – is something that should happen between the three of you – not just between mother and baby.

All this needs to be done quite consciously or else a pattern can be set up in which the father feels isolated and starts to drift away emotionally, opting out of involvement in any part of the domestic routine.

The new mother helps to link her partner with the baby and the matters of the home; in the same way the father can act as her link with the outside world when practical matters keep her confined. On a very basic level this means recognising that if she has been at home all day busy with the baby, she will feel a great need to be kept in touch with the world of adults. 'Real' conversation, rather than chit-chat is appreciated, as is proper attention for herself as a person, not just as the mother of the child.

If the new mother is having trouble adjusting to being at home after having worked, her partner's attitude to the change in her situation is also important. She loses the sense of herself as someone who does a job well (perhaps also feeling that she doesn't do this new job of looking after a baby quite so well!). Many men prefer their wives to stay at home and look after the children, but forget to show them the respect and appreciation they feel. The work of a full-time mother is expected yet undervalued in many parts of our society and even a woman who knows how important it is can be made to feel less interesting and useful than women in employment. Her partner's attitude is a vital element in reassuring her that this is not so and making her feel good about what she does.

Despite all of this, the birth of a child can ultimately bring you as close together as you originally hoped. Many couples hardly remember the upheavals brought about by their first child – or only do so with amusement – because they dealt with them so successfully.

INFERTILITY

Not being able to have children, or going through a period of infertility, is the cause of much distress to couples. The misery it brings affects the relationship profoundly, including (and especially) sex. It is rare for couples to seek counselling from Relate specifically for this problem, because attention is focused on the physical aspects of the issue. But agony aunts can confirm that the despair and unhappiness that couples experience is great, and that fertility problems make up a regular proportion of a problem page's mailbag. The letters ask for practical advice on the process of fertility investigations and treatment, but what shines through is the emotional anguish the couples feel. Few come to Relate with this difficulty because they feel that if a child is born the problems will vanish. This can be true, but meanwhile you need to look at the way what is happening affects your relationship.

With contraception so efficient most people concentrate on the issue of *not* having a baby until they are ready. Most couples assume that as soon as they want a child nature will take its course and they will conceive. But although 60 per cent of couples conceive within six months, the rest can take longer, and 15 per cent try for over a year before conceiving. Infertility is defined as the failure to conceive after a year of unprotected intercourse, and millions fall into this category.

Many go on to have children with or without fertility treatment, but meanwhile they will have worried about their prospects. Those who try to become pregnant for many years will find that to some degree their lives are shaped by this. Deciding to have a child, and trying for one, mean that you are emotionally preparing yourself for parenthood. This decision makes it difficult to take it lightly when month after month you discover that you are still not pregnant.

This is not just an issue for couples trying for their first child. Some couples have difficulty conceiving later on, and this can be just as distressing if you have strong ideas about how large your family should be, or if you were hoping to have children of both sexes.

‘——————— Talking point ————————

The intangible loss

Look at the box on grief and mourning on p.127. If you have been
told that you can never have children, you will grieve the loss, even
though no one has died. What has gone is the image you had of
yourself as a parent and the love you wanted to give to the children
you cannot have. Discuss your grief with your partner. For you,
the recovery stage will involve finding new meaning in life without
being a parent. Parenting takes up a relatively small proportion of
a couple's lives and all individuals need to find a purpose beyond
that of caring for children.

’

Your emotions

If you have been trying for a child long enough to be seeking medical help,
you have probably started on the long process of physical investigations.
We are not going to go into the details of the tests and treatments or
their alternatives here, but will instead concentrate on the emotional
side. This is particularly important because it is often ignored by the
doctors.

Infertile couples live with the anxiety that they may be unable to
bear a child. Those for whom this turns out to be true have to suffer the
grief of the loss and learn to come to terms with their infertility. The
investigations themselves cause stress, and some fear that too much
stress might harm their relationship.

Some of the pain stems from the fact in our society parenthood is
taken for granted. It is generally felt that having children is a natural
consequence of getting married. Couples will be asked when they plan to
start a family even before they are married – and still more so
afterwards. If you don't have children people assume that it's because
you have decided not to.

As time goes on and you don't conceive, you can start to feel a
failure. If you tell other people your problem they feel awkward – they
don't know what to say or they say the wrong thing. Many people give
uninformed advice ('just relax and it will happen'), or unwelcome comfort
('you're better off without children really'). Nothing outsiders can do or
say is going to make you feel better about it, and you can feel distanced
even from good friends. You might feel extra pressure if your own family
seems disappointed – particularly parents who have made it clear that
they are longing for grandchildren.

Just as distressing is that many other decisions must temporarily be deferred when you decide to have children: when and whether to move – into a larger place or not; career decisions for the woman, who might be wondering whether it is worth taking promotion or changing jobs if she is soon to become a mother. When months stretch into years without a pregnancy, it can feel as though your life is on hold and you are just marking time.

Problems with conception can originate with the man or the woman, or with both. In about 35 per cent of couples the woman has the problem and in an equal number of cases the problem stems from the man. For the remaining 30 per cent the problem is a joint one. Whoever has the actual difficulty, the problem remains joint, but it affects men and women slightly differently.

● **The woman's feelings.** A woman who wants a child is under even stronger pressures than a man who does. Girls and women learn that they are potential mothers, and this fact is incorporated in the image they build of themselves. Most women have a vague idea that 'some day' they will bear a child. It is married women – more so than their husbands – who are asked when they are going to have children or why it is that they don't have them.

In our society women are still given to understand that they can count being a 'good wife and mother' as primary goals and that paid work or a successful career are additional to this role. Even women who value their working lives tend to feel that children will make them more complete.

Because mothering involves profound changes in women's lives, coming to terms with the fact that you might never have children means altering your ideas about your future and shakes your image of yourself as a feminine woman. For women there is also the time factor: a man can father a child into old age, but sometime around her middle years a woman becomes infertile for good.

Once started on a fertility programme of tests and cures, it is also the woman who bears the brunt of the investigations and treatment, which are intrusive and sometimes distressing. This is hard to handle when you are already feeling sensitive.

● **The man's feelings.** Coming to terms with not being able to have children carries the same feelings of grief and loss for men. The difference is that in general a man's image about himself is not so bound up with parenthood: children are a welcome addition, rather than a central issue. But it does have an impact on a man's idea of himself as a sexual being. Many men equate fertility with sexual potency. A man who tries to have children but can't feels that his sexuality is called into question.

Your relationship

These feelings are bound to affect your relationship. If one of you is clearly the source of the problem you will feel a mixture of guilt and personal sorrow. The other partner can feel angry, however unreasonable this might seem. An unspoken issue might be, should the fertile partner find someone else – does he or she secretly want to?

Sometimes only one of you wants the child badly. This is also a source of tension as the other begins to feel that the issue of a child is more important to you than the relationship itself.

Talking all these matters through is vital. It won't be comfortable because of the powerful emotions involved, and if one of you feels it much more strongly than the other it won't be easy for either of you. You need to confront and explode the myths that your sexuality or your femininity are bound up with the ability to have children, and by so doing you will gain a better sense of your individuality and your relationship.

Whether you eventually have children or not, you still have to take care of your relationship. It is important to remember the reasons that brought you together in the first place; few relationships are formed only to have children, and the slice parenthood takes out of your lives is relatively short compared to today's life spans. Ultimately you have to function as a couple beyond your roles as parents.

While waiting to become parents – and even if you are never able to have children – you can afford to be more creative in your relationship than couples who are tied by the practical details of parenthood. Developing interests that you can share strengthens the bond between you, and you can also be more flexible in taking personal time alone. Couples whose lives are not centred on children can have more time to give to friendships and the all-round quality of their lives. Time spent putting effort into your relationship and into enjoying life now is never wasted. If you do have children they will have parents whose relationship has the stability that comes when love has been tested.

! ══════════════════ **Task** ══════════════════

Without children we could . . .

Make a list of the kinds of things you can only do if you don't have children and all the practical and financial considerations that they involve. Write down everything you can think of, even ideas that seem unrealistic. There is always something, even if it is 'go out in the evening without a babysitter'. Select two of the more possible choices and resolve to do them soon.

!

'—————————— Talking point ——————————

If we don't have a baby . . .

Discuss what you will do if it proves impossible to conceive a baby with your partner. Are you interested in the options of adoption or fostering, have you looked into surrogacy or Artificial Insemination by Donor? How would both of you feel about these? What are the practical problems and the benefits?

'

Sex

Trying for a baby will obviously have an impact on your sex life whether you are undergoing fertility treatment or not. In our society sex is usually far removed from conception: it has come to mean expressing your love for each other or trying to get maximum sensual and erotic pleasure from the act.

Sex can be particularly loving and exciting when you are hoping that it will result in a baby. But as the months go by without a pregnancy your attitude to sex is bound to undergo a change. As you grow more fixated on the idea of conceiving, sex can become more mechanical and goal oriented: the man must ejaculate, preferably at the time the woman is most fertile. Sex in other ways, at other times, or sex that doesn't result in a baby, may not seem worthwhile.

Once you start on a fertility programme of tests and treatment, your sex life can seem hijacked. Sex has to be performed at a particular time in particular ways, and sometimes the woman must go straight in for further tests after making love.

Sex that is programmed like this is bound to lose some of its appeal. Desire is a sensitive barometer to your sexual feelings generally and it is fuelled by erotic imaginings and the right conditions. It stands to reason that if sex has become purely the route to conception, and is timetabled by an outside authority, much of your natural desire to make love can go. Men can find it difficult to perform to order, and both of you might find it disconcerting that the woman must often initiate sex as she becomes trained to recognise the best time for her own body. Couples find that they are prepared to let much of the fun and pleasure in their sex life go by the board – as long as the man ejaculates it might as well be over quickly and efficiently.

While you are focused on conception you have to be prepared for the fact that sex is likely to seem more of a chore than a pleasure. Couples who come through this period best bring their sense of humour into play, but even this can be difficult when each month brings a disappointment that becomes increasingly hard to bear.

What is important to remember during this time is that it won't last forever. Either you will eventually succeed in becoming pregnant, or you will have to learn to come to terms with the fact that you will not have children. Either way, once you have stopped looking on every act of love as potentially making a baby you can start to rebuild your sex life into something that is pleasurable and satisfying again.

It is common, for a variety of reasons, for most couples to hit a low in their sexual relationship and temporarily lose desire for each other or for sex generally. As we saw in the preceding section, this can happen after the birth of a baby as well as at other times. It helps to realise that other couples go through phases such as this even when conception has not been an issue.

A large section of the chapter on Sex concentrates on loss of desire because it is so common. Reading it can help you once you are ready to deal with satisfaction in your sex life. Improving your sex life requires effort – though not unpleasant effort! – but that is the same for any couple in a long-term committed relationship.

If desire does not return, the issue is usually more complicated. Perhaps one or other of you is still harbouring angry or disappointed feelings that have not been fully expressed and handled. As with any unresolved issues in a relationship, they need to be aired in order for your relationship to continue to progress healthily and rewardingly.

AFFAIRS

An affair is what most people think of as *the* crisis in a relationship. For many the idea of their partners becoming involved with someone else is their greatest fear.

'Affair' covers a wide range of situations, from the one-night stand to the relationship that lasts for years. Most people think of an affair as a sexual relationship, but some people are also disturbed by friendships with an emotional rather than sexual closeness. By affair we mean any relationship with a third person that threatens the existing relationship between a couple. That is to say, even if one of you considers the outside relationship unimportant, it counts if your partner is unhappy about it and it causes you to re-evaluate your relationship.

The end of your relationship

It is usual to say that if your partner has an affair it will mean the end. In practice, though, the majority of people stay together after the discovery of an affair. Later we will look in detail at what characterises the relationships that stay together rather than split up. Briefly, what counts is what the affair means to both of you and how you handle the aftermath.

There is, however, a sense in which the relationship ends even when you stay together successfully and happily. The old relationship that you had *has* gone forever. If you stay together you are embarking on a relationship that has to be modified so much that it counts as a new one: the affair changes you both and therefore changes the relationship. Because of this counsellors treat an affair like a bereavement: the old relationship has died and needs to be mourned. For the new relationship to proceed healthily, both of you must recognise this, and therefore go through the stages of grief that accompany loss. Of course, some affairs are less important to both of you, and the accompanying emotions are less strong. But when it has been a major crisis in your life you can expect the impact to be greater.

Ruth and Lewis are an example of a couple for whom the suffering caused by an affair improved their relationship and their feelings about themselves. They were in their late twenties and had been married for eight years, with two children, aged seven and five.

Ruth, who had recently gone back to work as a helper in a children's nursery, was the one who had the affair. The man was much older, in his late forties, and was a delivery man who brought supplies to the nursery. He too was married with children, and after a short affair they both agreed to leave their families and set up home together. Within days the other man had gone back to his wife, and Ruth had no choice but to return to Lewis. Ruth was now deeply sorry about what she had done – 'something' had come over her to make her act in this way. She now wanted to make her marriage work.

Lewis was a computer engineer, occupying a junior position in his firm. He was a mouse – his own description – and it was his gentle quietness that had attracted Ruth to him originally. She was a bright, attractive girl, and he had not been able to believe his luck when she agreed to marry him.

During counselling a clear picture of their backgrounds and their relationship emerged. Both of them had had trouble relating to their same-sex parent. Lewis loved but feared his domineering father, who bullied his children. He had always vowed he would be different, and whenever he felt strong emotions he controlled them for fear that they would burst out in violent aggression, as had been the case with his father. He described himself as a mouse self-deprecatingly; secretly he was proud of it. Ruth was ashamed of her mother, who had kicked Ruth's drunken father out and had then proceeded to bring home a succession of men, occasionally going off to live with the latest lover. Ruth was mildly sexually abused by an uncle, which had made her wonder if she had 'asked for it' and reinforced her growing fear that deep down she was like her mother and would behave in the same way.

Lewis had attracted her because he was a nice, quiet, steady man who made few demands on her, even sexually. Both of them found shelter from their fears of being like their parents in their own relationship. Ruth was able to deny her sexual side and enjoy contentment as a housewife and mother – Lewis became one of her children. Lewis was able to abdicate responsibility to Ruth and arrange matters so that he never felt the strong emotions of which he was afraid.

But then Ruth started to feel restless. The man she had an affair with was persistent and seductive; she felt unable to put him off, as if she was no longer in control of herself.

The affair therefore brought them both face to face with their deepest fears. Ruth felt that it proved that she was like her mother and would respond to any man who made advances. Lewis was struggling for the first time with such strong and vengeful anger that he was terrified of what he might do.

When they arrived for counselling Lewis was desperately trying to hang on to his identity as a mouse. But, he said, the affair had roused him. What would he destroy if he let the anger out? His biggest fear was that he would turn into the kind of father his own was and harm his children emotionally and physically.

The counsellor helped them see that their choices were wider than either becoming like their parents or being the direct opposite. They could use the feelings that they feared constructively. Ruth did not have to deny her sexuality until it was drawn out by someone else, and Lewis had the choice of channelling his anger into constructive self-assertiveness rather than aggression.

Over the weeks, Lewis seemed to grow up before the counsellor's eyes. One session marked the turning point. He had told the counsellor that his mildness at work had caused his superior to put him down and promote other less able people over his head. He began the session by telling the counsellor that he had challenged his superior and put in a reasoned argument for promotion.

Almost immediately Lewis had been promoted, and he was promoted once again before the counselling finished: his salary went up by a third. The gain in confidence was immediate as Lewis realised that he had used his anger as a driving force and it had been beneficial rather than harmful. The impact on their family life was profound. Lewis became more assertive sexually and Ruth was able and willing to respond. Lewis also found that when the fear of his own anger went, so his relationship with his children – already good – improved. He felt more comfortable, capable and loving with them now that he had faced up to his anger and it hadn't made him into a tyrant like his father. Before the end of counselling Lewis made an appointment to see Ruth's lover and was able to express his anger and warn him off without losing control.

Ruth was delighted by the man Lewis was becoming. She no longer took all the burden of responsibility for the family. Sex was satisfying and pleasurable for the first time, and she was able to enjoy it without guilt. By the time they left counselling they had a fully adult relationship. About a month later the counsellor received a bunch of flowers from them with a note saying that matters were continuing to improve and they were very happy.

This was a particularly satisfying case for the counsellor, who knew that it was the willingness to face their problems – and to make changes – that helped Ruth and Lewis come through so well.

Why affairs happen

When an affair is revealed, one of the partners – usually the one who has just found out – sometimes says that it 'came out of the blue'. But this is rarely the case. Daily life brings most of us into contact with attractive people, and in a sexually free society it is not hard to find the opportunities to do something about it. These opportunities are usually resisted. Most affairs, even casual ones, happen because of problems within the relationship that are not being handled, making one of you more open to the idea of an affair.

The following are some of the main reasons that people already in a committed relationship seek someone else at a critical moment. Some point to serious problems, others to the fact that something is missing, but it might not even be anything major:

● **Protest.** There are times when one of you can feel positively entitled to have an affair. If you are rowing a lot over money or other issues to do with living together and home becomes fraught rather than a restful haven, being with someone else somewhere else might seem your right.

● **Insecurity.** If a partner feels rejected for some reason (as a man might if he loses the main focus of his partner's attention during pregnancy, or while she is caring for young children, or a woman might do if the man is wrapped up in his work) he or she might look for attention or closeness from someone else. So might someone who is feeling vulnerable about his or her age or waning sexual attractiveness: only the excitement of a new relationship and the admiration in the eyes of someone new can seem like proof that all is still well.

• **Sex and 'love'.** If one of you has gone off sex, or neither of you can be bothered to concentrate on anything but the most perfunctory sexual consummation, or sex just seems dull, an affair can seem the answer.

Perhaps you are seeking the kind of love we talked about in the first chapter, not recognising that the 'in love' feeling of being totally wrapped up sexually and emotionally in another person is transitory, part and parcel of the early days of a relationship. When that goes you might think that something has gone wrong, and start to look for it elsewhere.

In most of these cases it is what is sometimes called the 'fun' that is missing from the relationship.

The true one-night stand, a one-off that happens in extraordinary circumstances, can be a case of sexual curiosity, and is usually the only kind of affair that means nothing to you. But it can still hurt your partner, and can have an impact even if your partner doesn't find out if it leaves you feeling guilty towards him or her.

• **Growing apart.** As we have seen, couples can grow apart and develop differently until they feel they no longer give each other what they need.

• **Breakdown of relationship.** One or both of you can feel the relationship is completely dead. An affair at this stage is often about lining someone else up so that you have somewhere to go when you walk out.

The following reasons are why some people are 'affair prone', and continue to have affairs throughout a committed relationship, although they usually have no intention of breaking it up:

• **Excitement.** Some people recognise that the heady, exciting feelings of first love don't last, but they are hooked on them. They don't want to leave the steady partner, so go for a series of affairs or one-night stands. These are usually exciting: snatched, clandestine meetings with the focus on sex, plus the intoxication of finding, once more, someone who thinks you are wonderful and whom you can't wait to see.

• **Fear of intimacy.** Some people find the intimacy of a committed relationship hard to handle. An affair becomes a way of creating distance and privacy. Some people in long-term affairs, which are also apparently committed in their way, have, in effect, two part-time relationships – thereby preventing either having full intimacy.

People who find it easy to maintain emotional distance – indeed, who prefer it – can be puzzled at the pain caused by the discovery of their affair.

Effects of an affair

Whatever the reason behind it, the affair will affect the primary relationship whether it is discovered or not, because of the secret, separate life of the partner who is having the affair. An affair is not the solution to any of the above problems, it just defers one being reached. Postponing dealing with a problem means that it is likely to become worse, even though it might feel better for a while because of the distraction provided by the affair. When an affair is discovered you have to confront what caused it to happen. Your willingness to do so is what makes the difference to the eventual outcome.

For instance, one counsellor recalls Janine, who came alone for counselling after she had had an affair. Janine had set out to have the affair. She had been married for ten years and her relationship with her husband was good in all ways except for sex. Her husband said she was frigid and unresponsive, and as he had been her only lover she wondered if this was true. She approached a colleague at work, an older man, and told him her problem. He agreed to have a brief affair with her. This was arranged without difficulty. Janine enjoyed the sex and found she was normally responsive. The affair ended with good feelings on both sides. But what was Janine to do with what she had learnt? She came for counselling for weeks, during which she sorted out much of her feelings – but she was adamant she would not tell her husband about the affair, or even that she was coming for counselling. Before she left, she said that she would try to make changes in their sex life in a subtle way without her husband realising what had happened. Whether she succeeded or not the counsellor never heard. But she felt that it would be hard for Janine to make the necessary changes in such a circumspect way. If she had tackled the sexual problem by asking her husband to join her for counselling or sex therapy, rather than by having an affair, the problem could have been confronted head-on and more successfully.

Surviving the affair

Surviving the affair – and coming through to a newly stable and sometimes happier relationship – happens in two stages. There is the immediate impact when the affair is confessed to or discovered, a crisis time when many feelings are brought to the surface. During this period it can be impossible to tell what the outcome will be. It is followed by a time of sorting out, which includes understanding the function of the affair within the marriage and its importance to each partner, as well as discovering the commitment and ability of both partners to make the relationship change into something more stable and enduring.

The immediate impact

As we have seen, the discovery of an affair marks the end of the old relationship, and with that comes grief. Initially, it is the partner who has found out about the affair who feels this most immediately and strongly, though as the other partner begins to feel the impact of the changes in the relationship, his or her grief can follow on later.

Grieving

Grief is always painful, and mourning has a number of well-defined stages.

The first is shock and numbness and can last hours or days, when everything seems like a dream and you might be forgetful and feel 'out of it'. It is followed by the stage of yearning for what you have lost. This is the most emotionally violent stage, accompanied, as it can be, by outbursts of misery, intense anger and jealousy. This stage also includes disbelief and restlessness as the truth sinks in. After this comes disorganisation and despair. Your life has changed and it can throw you into depression and apathy as you find yourself unable to operate under the new conditions. The final phase, that of reorganisation, often alternates with the depression and despair, but you are now more able to examine the new situation you find yourself in and can start to think of ways of dealing with it. This includes the uncomfortable process of redefining yourself and your partner as well as your relationship, and it can still be painful. But it is also the turning point. It means you have put behind you thoughts of things getting back to what they were. With this realisation plans for the future can be made, and although this too is stressful, the result can be renewed happiness.

Coming to terms with an affair and rebuilding your relationship is not easy. There can be periods of darkness and hopelessness before you begin to see the light again. Some people do not move on and become stuck in one of the mourning phases – often the one of anger and jealousy, or depression and apathy. But if you successfully negotiate these stages you can find your relationship in better shape than it was before.

The second stage of anger, misery and jealousy usually follows quickly after the shock and numbness of the first stage. This is the opportunity to air uncomfortable emotions and deal with them.

Jealousy

Jealousy is at its most acute when you find out that your partner has been unfaithful. Most people experience jealousy physically as well as emotionally, sometimes as a pain in their guts.

Jealousy in these circumstances has two forms: sexual jealousy, and jealousy about the emotional closeness that has been shared.

In counselling it usually emerges that it is the emotional closeness that hurts for longest: people seem more able to get over jealousy when the encounters have been purely sexual. Where there has been emotional closeness there is more of a sense of betrayal. How much love was felt for the lover? Did they talk about you?

Jealousy is worsened if the lover was a friend or relation of yours, a situation that is not uncommon. This makes for a double betrayal, and feelings of jealousy and loss over both relationships.

Jealousy can last for a very long time, even when the affair is well and truly over, and the partner who was unfaithful has no intention of doing it again. Trust has gone and suspicion has taken over. Later on we look both at ways of overcoming this and how trust must be redefined in the relationship. Sometimes the wronged partner's jealousy lasts many years and becomes extreme and irrational. Looking at the section on jealousy in the chapter on Communication can help (see page 90).

Anger

Alongside the jealousy comes anger, and these emotions feed each other. The anger can be felt for many reasons and can be directed towards many people. These are the most common:

• **Anger at your partner.** There are a number of elements to this. Anger is obviously felt because of what your partner has done. But anger is also felt because your partner has turned out to be different to what you imagined and needed. When your partner behaves in a way that has deeply hurt you, or has acted on impulses of which you were not aware, he or she has become a subtly different person, temporarily a stranger until you have come to terms fully with what this means about your partner's nature. Being deceived, therefore, includes the deception involved in someone hiding aspects of his or her personality or desires, and this makes you angry. Lastly, anger at your partner is triggered by the fact that the person you would naturally look to for support is the very person who has caused you pain. If you have come to rely on your partner to look after you emotionally and give you security this is particularly hard.

• **Anger at the lover.** It is natural to feel anger at the lover. You can feel that this person has taken your partner away, or your partner might tell you that it was the lover who made all the running in the affair. Why didn't the lover back off, knowing about you and perhaps any children you have?

Although it is natural, this is the least effective outlet for your anger. If you concentrate your anger exclusively on the lover, it allows you to ignore your partner's role in the affair. It also makes it harder to confront your own part in the situation and any existing relationship problems that made the affair a possibility. Many people direct all their anger on the lover, with fantasies of revenge or actual physical attack.

● **Anger at yourself.** This can take a number of forms. Some people blame themselves totally for what has happened, particularly those who have taken all the emotional responsibility in the relationship. The affair can seem a failure of yours. Of course, this is as unfair as only blaming your partner or the lover. While it is healthy to examine what part you might have played in the problem, it is never entirely your fault. The person who has the affair is running away from the problem – whatever it is – and any blame should be shared equally. You can also feel angry at yourself for being so blind or stupid and taking so long to recognise what was happening, or for acting in ways that made the affair possible.

● **Anger at others.** You can feel angry at anyone else who knew about the affair. Sometimes you are angry because others knew and did not tell you. You can be equally angry at anyone who knew and passed on the information. Whether your anger is rational or irrational, it is natural. It has to be faced before it will go away.

Fear and misery

In this emotionally turbulent time you will also be very unhappy, and that sadness is often mixed with fear. The fear can be about losing your partner and becoming single again, with all the changes that would mean. The fear is also to do with the changes in you and your partner and the unknown impact they will cause even if you stay together.

These emotions are always strong, but they can be sharper if you have relied on your partner for all your emotional needs, or have largely defined yourself through your relationship. When this prop seems to have been taken away, or it is changing, you have to look to yourself for strength, which you might not be sure you have.

Dealing with the strong emotions

There is only one way for these strong and painful emotions to be dealt with healthily, and that is to talk them through. This also means talking about the affair (or series of affairs) and the lovers involved.

Talking about these matters is never easy for either of you, but it is often the person who had the affair who is most reluctant to do so.

Guilt can stop that person wanting to talk about the affair, as can grief and loss connected to the affair being over, and can make him or her want to try to forget about what happened. Some people don't want to talk about the affair because they say it was not important. But it *is* important because of the impact it has on the partner and the relationship. However difficult, these issues must be aired. Both of you need to understand the depth of the *hurt* that has been caused. Not talking about this usually means that only the *anger* is expressed.

The need of the wronged partner to talk about what has happened goes beyond the need to express the emotions concerned. He or she also has to make sense of what has happened and why. When it comes as a complete surprise this can take quite a long time. People are compelled to rehash constantly any major happening in their lives until they can come to terms with it – as you do after someone has died, when you relive the last days and hours, wondering if anything could have been done differently, or as a woman needs to talk through the experience of giving birth many, many times.

This, of course, includes wanting to know what the lover was like. These questions – and the answers – might seem only to produce pain. But they are part of the process of understanding. Knowing what the lover was like is useful in trying to define what the affair meant to the relationship and what gap it was filling.

This can be exasperating for the person who had the affair, and can seem pointless and perhaps punishing. He or she must understand that not talking about it is unbearable for the other partner, and that this apparently obsessive interest in details and events helps in the healthy process of putting it behind him or her.

The partner who had the affair needs to answer the questions honestly. Nothing you say will be worse than what your partner imagines if you don't answer or are evasive. People only continue with relentless questioning if they sense that the truth is being withheld or distorted. It might seem kinder to play down the significance of the affair, but your partner is likely to sense that you are doing this and therefore continue to harass you. If you succeed in not talking about what has happened, your partner's anxiety will increase and the unanswered questions will continue to cause their own pain.

The more you can talk through what has happened, the more likely you are to move on to the next stages and achieve a satisfactorily rebuilt relationship. When this airing of the details of the affair is allowed to take the time it needs there will come a moment when it naturally stops. Talking it through, and thereby both coming to understand why the affair happened, means you are more likely to make changes that will stop such a thing happening again. If you ignore the issues the fundamental problem remains, and with that the likelihood of it all happening again.

!══════════════════ *Task* ══════════════════

Having your say

When one of you has had an affair, the other is going to feel full of bitterness and anger about what has happened. Talking about it is one of the best ways of dealing with these emotions until they have run their course. If you find this difficult to do without arguing, the following solution often helps:

Pick a time once a week during which the one who has not had the affair can talk for one hour, saying everything he or she wishes to about what it means to him or her.

The pact is that the subject is not mentioned at other times, as long as the person who had the affair listens fully without interrupting, contradicting or arguing. This is not an interrogation but a chance to vent any feelings fully. This time should be set aside every week until the person doing the talking decides to call a halt. Couples who do this properly often find that it does not take too many weeks before the partner has said everything he or she wishes to say.

!

The function of the affair

Talking fully and frankly about your feelings and about the affair makes it more possible to understand the underlying reasons why it happened. These are the categories into which reasons are likely to fall:

● **Getting out of the relationship.** Sometimes it quickly becomes clear that the function of the affair has been to help you leave the relationship. In this case, when your partner finds out, you leave for the lover – or you might decide to leave both of them. In this case you are usually not willing to work with your partner to mend the relationship, but just want it to end. More often, though, the affair has a less radical purpose:

● **Filling a gap in the relationship.** Rather than confront whatever difficulties there are in the relationship, you use the affair to make you feel better about it, or distract you from the problems. When you tell your partner about it, or make it easy for your partner to find out, it is usually your subconscious way of drawing attention to the problems or of expressing your dissatisfaction or hostility.

When you have no intention of letting your partner find out, it sometimes means that only minor things are missing from your relationship: sex might be less fun than previously, you might be going through a period of dullness or irritation, or you might be getting on less well with your partner. Surveys into when people are most likely to have affairs show that the most vulnerable time is the period of disillusionment we discussed in the first chapter, after the 'in love' feelings have faded, when usually there is nothing seriously wrong with the relationship.

When affairs that start out like this go on for a long time, or you develop the habit of always having an affair 'on the go' even though the lovers vary, then the affair has a more important function in the relationship. The affair becomes a prop, allowing you to ignore the fundamental problems and weakening the primary relationship.

! ——————————— *Task* ———————————

Talking it through

When one of you has had an affair and you both want to put it behind you, it is necessary to talk about it and what it meant. To do this effectively and healthily you need some ground rules.

Rule 1. Use 'I messages', as explained in the chapter on Communication: talk about how events make you feel, but don't blame.

Rule 2. Only ask questions if you are prepared to listen to the reply. Questions such as 'Did you love him/her?', 'What's wrong with our relationship?' could produce answers that are upsetting. Don't interrupt before your question has been answered.

Rule 3. Don't attack if you don't get the answer you want to hear. Remember that your partner can't control *feelings*, only *behaviour*.

Rule 4. Answer questions honestly. If you don't know the answer, say so – but don't hide behind 'don't know' if you really do know.

Rule 5. If it turns into an argument, stop. You won't get anywhere that way.

Rule 6. If tempers run so high that you always find yourself arguing, reread the chapter on Communication to see where you are going wrong. Try to get rid of the unhelpful ways of communicating if you really want to sort matters out.

!

● **Acting as a prop to your marriage.** When there are grave problems in your marriage, or problems that have become grave because you have never been able to face them, the affair can, paradoxically, act as a stabilising influence.

This is often the case in relationships where convenience and convention are very important: for instance, you are married, and although you are not happy and the relationship is poor, you do not believe divorce is the answer; perhaps the relationship fulfills your need for security, comfort and support and you don't require anything else from it; or you have children and don't want to disrupt their family life. An affair or series of affairs means that you worry less about the unsatisfying aspects of your marriage because you are successfully finding them elsewhere. This means that you are less demanding of your partner and can live together almost happily.

Sometimes it is when a secret affair ends that the real cracks start to show in your marriage, because the unsatisfactory elements become harder to ignore.

An example of this is the case of Saul and Priscilla, who came for counselling when they had only been married for eight months. It was a curious case: they had had an affair for fifteen years, throughout Priscilla's marriage to Brian. Brian had died eighteen months previously and she had married Saul after the mourning period was over. Their affair had been ecstatic throughout the fifteen years, and Priscilla's marriage to Brian had been reasonably happy. But now that Brian was dead, it became apparent how essential a triangular relationship was to Priscilla. Saul became convinced that she had found someone else to be her 'other man', and his suspicions turned out to be true. Priscilla had a fear of confrontation and difficult emotions and found it impossible to say what she needed in a relationship. She could only cope by finding someone to balance what was lacking. She resisted counselling because she still could not bring herself to tell Saul what the relationship lacked and how it could be improved.

During the affair – the impact on the marriage

The longer the affair, or series of affairs, the more impact it has on the marriage. A one-off and short affair will still affect the relationship, but not as deeply or radically. These are the main ways the affair affects the marriage:

● **Loss of intimacy.** Intimacy and free communication can be disrupted by the lying that is necessary when you are having an affair. The longer the affair goes on the more damaging this is. If you have to watch what you say it puts distance between you and you lose the natural spontaneity of a frank relationship. It destroys true intimacy, because you must watch yourself in case you contradict something you've said previously.

Lying is not just a form of words. There are lies of omission – not saying where you've been or what you've been up to, or changing the subject if it becomes tricky.

● **Loss of quality.** If the affair is filling a gap in your marriage, or acting as a prop, you lose the urge to maintain the quality of your relationship. The contrast between the two relationships can be unfairly distorted in favour of the lover. If your snatched moments together are always happy, fun and exciting, and time with your partner is the normal mix of life, including rows and boredom, you may come to believe that it is your lover who is the more satisfying partner. Every row and petty irritation with your spouse can confirm this. The effect can be to make you withdraw further. The kinds of things people reserve to tell their partners – hopes, fears, jokes, and worries – now become shared with, or even exclusively saved for, the lover, weakening the ties between you and your spouse. Telling all the good things to your lover – when you feel positive, excited and happy, and saving only the miserable, down moments for your partner, can unbalance the relationship, making it gloomy and dispiriting. It therefore becomes true that your spouse 'doesn't understand' you, because you keep so much back.

● **Sex.** Your sex life isn't necessarily affected. Some people find it perfectly possible to maintain reasonable sexual relationships with two different people. But sex often does suffer: usually this is when your sex life at home has become unsatisfying, and rather than see what can be done about it you look for excitement in sex elsewhere.

Staying together

It is only when you have fully understood the significance and impact of the affair, and you have worked through your feelings about it, that you can make an informed decision about whether you want to stay together. This will involve adjustment and change. But first of all both of you have to want to stay in the relationship and both have to be prepared to make it work.

The one who had the affair

As we have seen, affairs broadly fall into two categories: the affair that happens because of dissatisfactions within a relationship that you want to maintain, and the affair that happens when you are mentally and emotionally preparing to leave the relationship.

Gloria and Dennis are an example of the second category. They had been married for six years and had two young children. They came for counselling initially because Gloria had gone off sex, and she didn't like Dennis to be near her. Dennis was in awe of Gloria, a pretty, athletic young woman, who attended dance classes three times a week. She said that she wanted to stay in the marriage so long as Dennis left her alone. Dennis had persuaded her to come for counselling because he wanted the problems with their sex life resolved.

The counsellor found their case very hard. Dennis seemed prepared to look closely at himself and the relationship and to put effort into making changes. Gloria, on the other hand, was resistant to everything and was not prepared to work at the relationship. On nights when she wasn't at the dance class she often went out with her girlfriends. There was never any time to give to Dennis. In the end the counselling reached stalemate and they stopped coming.

Six months later Dennis came back in a terrible state. Gloria had just left him. Throughout the counselling, she confessed, she'd been having an affair, and now she was moving in with the other man. The counsellor continued to see Dennis and helped him come to terms with what had happened. But there was no chance of Gloria returning. The resistance she had shown to counselling had been because she had already turned her back on the marriage, but had not been quite ready to leave.

On the other hand Jamie, who had had many affairs, was fundamentally committed to his relationship with Dawn. He was a very attractive man whose work often meant travelling. During these travels he invariably had brief affairs, but he always left obvious clues for Dawn to find – lipstick-stained handkerchiefs, love notes. During counselling it emerged that he had had a very difficult relationship with his domineering but neglectful mother. She only gave him attention when he was naughty, and then she would punish him severely. He hated the punishments but they were his only sign that his mother cared about him. He craved the approval and attention of women that the sexual encounters gave him and he viewed the disapproval of Dawn as proof that she cared.

It was no surprise to the counsellor that he had married a woman who looked the strong and domineering type. Dawn was big-built and competent. She appeared to play his mother, was strict and untender, and by letting her find out about his affairs he was constantly putting himself in the position where she was telling him off.

But Dawn was only outwardly like his mother. She was far nicer and much more vulnerable. She had put up with his affairs for as long as she could because she was scared of losing him, but she had reached the end of her tether. She had finally left Jamie because she couldn't take any more. Jamie had always tried to provoke a reaction from Dawn, but this one was stronger than he had bargained for. He initiated the counselling because he didn't want their marriage to end.

They looked at how the relationship had operated: Jamie needed Dawn to be strong – so she was. This unconscious collaboration stopped either of them from developing: Jamie didn't have to grow up and Dawn had to suppress her more tender side. The turning point came during one session when Dawn broke down and wept. Jamie had never seriously considered the hurt he was causing her – he had seen her anger but not her pain. For the first time he was forced to look at matters from Dawn's point of view; the realisation came to him that playing the naughty little boy was inappropriate and that Dawn had feelings and needs too.

When Dawn started to cry the counsellor offered her a handkerchief, but she turned down the offer abruptly: she had brought her own. This led to a discussion about Dawn's facade of strength which meant she would not allow herself to be helped. On a later occasion when she cried again, she shrugged Jamie off when he tried to put his arm round her. She came to see that by hiding her vulnerability she made it easier for him to act irresponsibly. Allowing her softer side to emerge meant that she would also be able to give Jamie the loving attention he sought from other women, which would mean he did not have to resort to his attention-grabbing tactics.

By the end of the counselling their relationship had moved to a point where Jamie could say quite confidently that he would not need his casual affairs. Because of the changes in both of them, Dawn knew that he meant it.

The wronged partner

The attitude of the wronged partner is also important. Some people don't want to continue with the relationship when they find out about the affair. Others want to do so – but their attitude to the affair and the reasons behind it are crucial if the marriage is to be rebuilt.

Most people blame the straying partner for the effect an affair has on the relationship. This is not the way it is regarded in counselling, where the affair is seen as the consequence of a relationship problem. It doesn't help to apportion blame, and it certainly is not easy – the complicated nature of a relationship means that both partners make a contribution to the situation, knowingly or unknowingly. If the wronged partner can't see this it can make for future difficulties.

Ken and Michelle are an example of this. Ken came for counselling on his own because he was four years into an affair with his secretary. His wife had just found out and he was now at a cross-roads. He didn't know whether to leave Michelle or try to make a go of his marriage. He was an astute and successful businessman who was out of touch with his emotions. He said that in his business life he was used to buying in outside expertise when he hit something he couldn't handle. He was treating Relate in the same way – as experts who could tell him what to do.

The counsellor had to make it clear that she was not going to tell him what he should do. Instead, she helped him explore his feelings about both women and his relationships with them. Over a few sessions he came to realise that the affair with his secretary was essentially a fantasy which would evaporate if they lived together full time. He ended it, and she left the job.

During the course of these sessions Ken had talked about the difficulties in his marriage. He painted a picture of Michelle as very dependent on him and lacking in confidence. There were numerous ways in which their relationship was very unsatisfactory, which is what had made him vulnerable to the charms of his kindly, attractive secretary. Now he and Michelle had decided to make a go of it he wanted her to come for counselling as well.

The first thing that struck the counsellor was how different Michelle was from the picture Ken had painted. She was quite strong, and controlling in a subtle way – she dominated Ken with an appearance of weakness. She was unable to see any reason why Ken should have had an affair. Essentially they were living different marriages: Ken had an image of Michelle that was quite at odds with the reality, and Michelle had an image of their marriage as being perfect until the other woman had appeared. Michelle was naturally angry, but the anger seemed to go further than the understandable emotions awakened by the knowledge of Ken's adultery.

The counsellor suspected that Ken's affair was his subconscious way of asserting himself against a strong and controlling wife and an unsatisfactory relationship. Michelle saw herself as the wronged wife – a victim of problems that had nothing to do with her. Beyond her anger there were no tender feelings for Ken, and she neither saw nor cared that he had been hurt.

When the counsellor tried to help them explore why Ken had had the affair and what might have been wrong with the marriage, Michelle maintained that there were no reasons. She felt that now the affair was over she wanted things to go back to the way they were before. Ken indicated that he wouldn't be happy with that. The counsellor gently pointed out that the relationship was changed anyway by the affair. Both of them seemed angry with the counsellor, Michelle, because she didn't like what was being said, and Ken because he felt she was failing in her 'expert's' role of making everything right. The counsellor likened counselling to undoing some knitting that had gone wrong until you found the mistake. It is only when you have done that that you can start to knit it up again. They were still at the unravelling stage.

They didn't come back for counselling, however. The counsellor felt that the difficulties were too deep-rooted and painful for Michelle to face up to. Initially, she thought, they might be united by their anger against her – but that would not last. Michelle's insistence on blaming Ken would mean that the essential problems in their relationship remained untouched.

The aftermath

Even when a couple decide to stay together and some of the more painful emotions have been dealt with, there is still work and some unhappiness to come.

The phase of disorganisation that we talked about – a normal stage of mourning – usually follows. There is reassessment for both of you. The partner who has had the affair has to find new ways of operating within the relationship without the safety valve of the affair, and this involves thinking in new ways about both him or herself and the partner. The other partner also uses this time to ask such fundamental questions as 'What do I now want for me, from life, from the relationship?' Both might be struggling with a sense of failure, as well as the depression and apathy that occasionally accompanies this kind of soul-searching.

As we have seen, it is those couples who are able to see that blame can not be apportioned who can move on faster and more healthily into a new relationship. A willingness to accept the changes that have occurred also helps.

The changes in both of you

Both of you have changed, and both of you have to relearn who the other is. Many people find hidden strengths when they discover that their partners have had affairs. As we have seen, when you have looked to your partner for emotional support in the past, you now have to find the strength in other ways and from within yourself. People who have been able to do this grow more independent. If this is your situation, you will feel very differently about your relationship. Things that previously you endured you are no longer prepared to accept, and you might find that there are certain things you now feel able to demand from your partner.

If you had the affair, and never seriously considered leaving your partner, you now have to confront a changed person. If your affair was a way of controlling your relationship – dissatisfactions and all – you can find your newly assertive partner disturbing.

You have changed too. By committing yourself to the relationship you have to be able to confront aspects of yourself and your life together that you have previously been able to ignore. This often means facing up to weaknesses or needs that you have never been able to put into words. By choosing to act in a responsible way you might find that parts of you that have remained adolescent now need to be allowed to grow up. If an affair allowed you to divide aspects of yourself between two people, you now have to learn how to show your complete self to one person. This is uncomfortable for you and also for your partner. Your partner can be surprised and disturbed by the new you, and if you seemed a tower of strength before, any vulnerability you now show can be unnerving.

Living with your changed relationship

These changes, although difficult to experience and manage, often result in a much better balanced relationship. If one of you has been able to tap previously buried strength, and the other is able to express the weaker, gentler side, you can now meet as equals in your relationship. If, while coping with the discovery of the affair, you make a genuine breakthrough in communication, the affair can be seen as the catalyst you needed to make your relationship better.

But some people can't cope with these changes or try to deny them. Other people seize on them to change the balance of power in the relationship in a negative way. Sometimes one of you might want to stay in the relationship only because you fear the alternative. Or the wronged partner might use the affair as a stick to beat the other one with. This means you continue together bitterly and unlovingly, or perhaps break up at a later date. Some people make a workable peace pact between them, which often means agreeing not to deal with the issues raised by the affair, and because of this they never become close again.

An affair that shakes everything up is an opportunity to make it better than before. You can merely survive and live unhappily – or you can survive healthily and positively. The choice is yours, and counselling can help. One area that has to change for the healthy process to be complete is your attitude towards trust.

Redefining trust

Many people say that the most important legacy of an affair is the loss of trust in your partner. Now you can never be sure that it won't happen again.

Trust is fragile: like a delicate ornament it can be broken in a moment, and although it can be patched up it will never be what it was. What is sometimes left when trust has been destroyed is constant suspicion, which can make a shaky relationship worse. Trust is likely to be partly regained if the straying partner has been completely honest about the affair. The less you have talked about it the more likely it is for the wronged partner to remain suspicious and untrusting.

But complete trust is not essential to a good relationship. Trust, in the sense that most people mean it, involves knowing someone so thoroughly that you can always predict how they will behave. It also means believing that they are 'yours' for life.

Neither of these two elements is realistic. As we have seen, you can never know another person better than very well – there will always be things you don't know – and people change over time so sometimes you know them less well than previously. Nor do you own anyone, partner or child. The affair has taught you the hard way that this is so.

So, this complete, unthinking trust must go. But what can emerge from the aftermath of an affair is a different sort of trust, ultimately more healthy and helpful: a commitment not to hurt each other or further risk the relationship. The more effort you both put into making something positive out of your relationship after the discovery of the affair the less likely it is that either of you will want to risk jeopardising it again.

Trust, in the old sense, ties up your feelings of security in your partner and the relationship. But true security is only to be found within yourself. If the affair has strengthened your sense of self and your independence you will find this to be so. More healthy than the old kind of trust is the development of a relationship that you want for itself. This is likely to happen if you both give time to your individual development. The better you feel about yourself and the more sure you are that you could survive without the relationship – yet *choose* to be in it – the better you are able to tolerate the separateness of your partner. What you can expect from your newly formed relationship is the acknowledgement that pain has been caused and that if you are to live contentedly together you should try to avoid it happening again.

If you have looked at the roles you have both played in making the affair possible, both of you will have realised that you have shortcomings. Accepting that these are normal human failings, and that it is unrealistic to expect perfection in each other or in the relationship, is important.

Ultimately respect and tolerance are more essential than trust. Respect and tolerance for each other's feelings and for each other as human beings make you require higher standards of behaviour from yourselves. When this happens trust ceases to be the important issue between you.

A DEATH IN THE FAMILY

When someone close to you dies you will feel grief and pain as well as other difficult emotions. We are not going to look in detail at coping with bereavement: appropriate organisations are mentioned in the Further help section. What concerns us is how the death of a relative affects your relationship. This it will do temporarily – but sometimes the effects are more profound. It is a time of such powerful emotions that inevitably other feelings – good and bad – become churned up.

When your relationship is good, weathering this time together can create a special closeness. But if things have not been going too well between you, the anguish of a bereavement can bring matters to a head. As we have seen, some couples avoid coping with problems in a relationship because they fear the upheaval and discomfort of change. But, as we will see later, the great pain and upheaval of coping with the death of a loved one can make you more daring about tackling the other problems in your life. The intense suffering of bereavement can make you feel that the lesser pain of examining what is wrong with your relationship is bearable. The changes caused by a death close to you can also make you more prepared to make the changes that will benefit your relationship. The case, in Chapter 1, of Alison and Mike, whose second child died soon after birth, is an illustration of this. This is not to say that a death is ever welcomed, but that you can use your suffering in a positive way.

! ——————————— *Task* ———————————

They are avoiding me

It is common for people who know you to feel embarrassed when you have suffered a death in the family. They don't know what to say or do and sometimes they take the easy way out by avoiding you.

This can cause you unnecessary misery if you believe it is because they don't care or are rude. Sometimes you decide that you don't want to have anything more to do with them.

Give them the benefit of the doubt, and don't take it badly. When you are feeling more up to seeing people, approach them yourself. It helps to give them guidelines about what you want from them, for instance, 'I need to talk about it', or 'You don't have to say anything', or 'I would appreciate some practical help' or 'I don't want to think or talk about it today'

!

Fear of death

Death is one of the last taboo subjects because almost everyone is frightened of the thought of it happening to those they love and to themselves. Counsellors say that most couples find it hard to discuss, particularly older couples or couples who have experienced an early death in their families.

Janet and Bill, a couple in their late sixties, came for counselling because Janet had recently become very jealous and they were arguing a lot. Janet said that Bill paid too much attention to other women at social evenings and she had become convinced that he was going to go off with someone else.

Through counselling it emerged that the real issue was loneliness, and underlying Janet's fear of Bill going off with another woman was her fear of him dying and leaving her alone. Many of their friends were widowed. Because it was a subject that they had been unable to discuss, Janet's fears had to emerge in a way that she felt able to express. Bill feared death, too, and this had made him act uncharacteristically flirtatiously with other women to bolster his feelings that he was fit and well. Talking about their fears of death during counselling brought them closer together. It did not take away their fears, but it removed the false tensions between them, and the jealousy and rows stopped.

Death of your parents

This is the most likely close death that you will experience as a couple. If family relationships have been good, it will not just be the child of the parents who grieves, but the partner too. If your parents die naturally of old age, you may well have to deal with a series of deaths in a short number of years.

Apart from grief, you will experience other feelings that affect your relationship. Your parents dying leaves you orphaned, whatever your age. Even if your relationship with them was not good, a subconscious part of you was aware that you had a 'mum and dad', to whom you were a child. With their passing the link to your childhood goes, and with that comes the feeling that you are next in line. Even if you never put these feelings into words they are powerful, and they cause you to reassess yourself at the same time as you are coping with grief.

Some people start to act in ways that seem strange to their partners. Someone whose parents were strong and controlling, and whose life was shaped by trying to please them, may now want to alter structures that were not of his or her choosing.

Sharing your grief (and all the other feelings that are thrown up) helps; locking them away can create a barrier between you. Quite often counsellors see couples who come with a relationship problem and find that there has been a recent bereavement. When this is properly talked through the relationship problem sometimes sorts itself out.

This was true with Belinda and Sean, who were having terrible rows because of Sean's inadequacy as a father. Belinda was angry about it and Sean was depressed about his failings. Now they were on the point of separating and so had come to Relate.

What the counsellor quickly discovered was that Belinda's father had died eighteen months before, and her mother had followed six months later. At exactly the same time, Sean's father had died. Both of them were struggling with tremendous feelings of loss and pain, but they had never talked to each other about it. Belinda's feelings were expressed through anger, and Sean's through icy withdrawal.

Much of the counselling focused on the bereavements. With the counsellor they both became able to express the mixed feelings of anger, guilt, loss and sorrow. This was a breakthrough for both of them, because they had never been in touch with their full range of emotions before. Belinda had always been the angry partner, and most of her other emotions had been buried or immediately consumed by anger. Sean had been brought up by women, most of whom had been powerful and angry too, and he had always withdrawn emotionally. Belinda's anger seemed quite natural to him, and he wasn't aware of how his habit of isolating himself emotionally made it worse.

Alongside this, the counsellor worked with Sean on practical ways of coping with his children. Sean's parents had divorced when he was young and he had grown up without his father around and had always felt that he had no personal knowledge of how a father should behave on a daily basis – his father had simply taken him out from time to time and bought him presents. Sean tried his best with his own children but often got it wrong. He usually overreacted: when his son expressed an interest in American football he went out and bought him the full gear. His son went off the idea and Sean felt rejected. His impulses towards his children were all kindly, but somehow they missed the point.

There was nothing very wrong with Sean's relationship with his children that confidence and certain adaptations wouldn't put right, and as the counselling progressed, both Belinda and Sean seemed to forget that this was what had brought them there in the first place. Both had calmed down now that they were dealing with the grief – the real cause of their strong emotions. Belinda discovered in herself a desire to go to university (her mother had always been disappointed that she had dropped out) and Sean supported her decision to do so.

As Sean allowed his bottled-up feelings to emerge, so too did his sense of humour and his long-lost adventurous spirit. He'd been a great traveller in his youth but he and Belinda hadn't been anywhere for years. Sean had recently developed a fear of any form of transport, but as the counselling went on this disappeared – it had been connected to his feelings about death. By the end of counselling their relationship had entered a new and very promising phase. They were talking more and both were able to express soft and sadder emotions, which brought them together. They fixed up to go abroad on holiday, and soon after the counsellor received a postcard from them. In the following year they went abroad twice more and sent her cards each time. The messages expressed excitement and happiness with the way their lives were progressing.

Reaching the age your parents were when they died

Many people who have successfully come to terms with their parents' deaths find a new anxiety emerging when they reach the age their parents were when they died – particularly the same-sex parent. This is the time when you are likely to start thinking more about your own death. Like any worry that is unacknowledged and unshared, it can affect your behaviour and your relationship. In counselling, when one or other partner is represented as suddenly behaving differently and out of character – giving up a job, or having an affair or becoming very anxious and depressed – it sometimes emerges that this new behaviour started at around the age the same-sex parent died. When the feelings this caused are looked at the other behaviour often becomes more understandable.

Death of children

When one of your children dies you suffer the most acute form of grief. You experience the pain that comes when anyone you love dies, but this is worsened by the feeling that it is unnatural for your child to die before you, and you also have all the anger and guilt that often goes along with this. It is among the most difficult experiences a couple ever has to endure. When you are both suffering so deeply it can be hard for you to give each other comfort, and some couples avoid each other at this time, as we saw in Chapter 1 with Alison and Mike – when their baby died he escaped by having an affair.

Anger always accompanies grief, but when it is a child who dies this is intensified: you blame yourself, each other, the doctors, fate. It is understandable that the violence of these feelings spills over into your relationship.

The same powerful feelings are thrown up when you have suffered a miscarriage. Outsiders often feel that this is not the same, as you never knew the child who died. But anyone who has experienced a miscarriage knows that the grief is just as strong.

This was the case with Douglas and Jenny. Douglas initially came on his own for counselling. He was 25 and Jenny was 24. They had two children under five. He complained that their relationship was a disaster. Their sex life had ceased and she never talked to him.

When Jenny joined them for counselling an essential fact left out by Douglas emerged: Jenny had had a miscarriage a few months previously. The doctor had been negligent and Douglas was pursuing a claim against him.

Both of them were angry. Jenny's anger became focused on Douglas because she wanted to deal with her sadness and didn't want the added pressure of taking action against the doctor. Douglas's anger was focused on the doctor and also on Jenny because her anger made her withdraw from him sexually and emotionally. When they were able to work through their grief and anger and stopped taking it out on each other, it was revealed that certain long-standing problems had been brought to a head.

They had always had difficulty in saying to each other what they felt and needed. This had resulted in a multitude of grievances that were never talked about. Each resented the other for not realising what the problems were. Communicating about their deep sorrow helped free them to talk about the other issues. Counselling was then able to progress and they dealt with all the problems, including the sexual one.

In Douglas and Jenny's case the feelings aroused by the miscarriage made a previously unsatisfactory relationship unbearable. They were already so emotionally vulnerable because of the miscarriage, that when they came for counselling they were more open to the kinds of self-analysis it demanded. This was even more strikingly so with Henrietta and Chris.

Chris had forced Henrietta to come for counselling because he couldn't take their relationship any longer. Over three sessions a picture of their marriage emerged. Henrietta bullied Chris, and he emotionally rejected her. Sex was very infrequent and unsatisfying. Henrietta hated it, but she took control of it. It was only when matters were at their worst between them that she would allow sex. Chris would know that it was 'the night' because she would put on perfume and the same low-cut dress. He would react with great excitement and try to get her to cuddle and show him some affection. She would brush him away irritably and they would argue, but when they went to bed she would allow him to make love to her. Henrietta would simply let it happen, distracting herself with thoughts of other things. This had been going on for the eighteen years of their marriage. They had a twelve-year-old son.

Counselling did not progress. They each wanted the other to change. Neither could see what they were doing wrong. Henrietta was bitterly resentful that they were talking about such matters to a counsellor at all.

Then the unimaginable happened: their son was killed in an accident. The counsellor expected them to cancel counselling, but they wanted to continue. Throughout the next few months they lived through the horror of their grief. It was a terrible time, but the extraordinary side effect was that they stopped being defensive about themselves and began to be able to look at the way they had each contributed to their sterile, unhappy marriage. It was as though, said the counsellor, because they felt they had lost what mattered most to them they had nothing else to lose. The grief brought to the surface a host of other emotions, and the insights they gained into their marriage came much more quickly than is usually the case.

The pain of their grief didn't lessen, but for the first time they felt emotionally close, and they could really support each other. The barriers were down, and because of this Henrietta began to feel differently about sex. Their relationship, which hadn't seemed to stand a chance, looked as if it was now going to become something worthwhile.

Coping with death

Grief in all its stages has to be endured and lived through. Read through the box on grief and mourning on p.127 if you are not sure what the stages are.

If one of you is grieving much more than the other (your parent has died, for instance) the other has a chance to show how supportive he or she can be. It needs patience and compassion, because grieving takes the time it takes, and although the emotionally violent stages might be over within months, the rest of the healing process can take much longer.

! ─────────────── *Task* ───────────────

I wanted to tell you . . .

When someone dies one of the painful elements is not being able to talk to that person any more. Everyone has things they wished they had said. Write a letter to your loved one who has died – even if it is a baby you have lost – saying all the things that are in your heart, and put it in a safe place.

!

• **Talk about it.** Talking and listening are very important throughout all the stages of grief. Talking helps you come to terms with what has happened, and you will often find it necessary to go over and over the same ground. This repetition is important as it is one of the best ways of helping the truth to sink in. It is wrong to think that talking about it just 'rakes it up' and that it is better to forget it. Forgetting is impossible, and people who are grieving have a need to talk. The partner just needs to listen – words are unnecessary and sometimes unhelpful – and to offer comfort and support, helping in practical ways and taking the pressure off the bereaved person.

If you both are bereaved, you need to share your feelings and thoughts, including the uncomfortable ones of anger and guilt. It is harder to come to terms with your loss if you don't talk about it, and it is also unhelpful. Some of the stronger emotions will then boil up and be displaced. As we have seen, angry feelings can be taken out on your partner when they are really about something else. If you let your anger out without examining the guilt and hurt beneath it you risk causing a problem between you or making existing problems worse. Looking at the section on anger in the chapter on Communication can help.

MOVING

Few couples would rate the experience of moving as traumatic enough to be a crisis that will profoundly shake their relationship. However, as it is very stressful it is worth looking at briefly here. It is important to bear in mind that it can cause you an uncomfortable few months, even if you are moving to a better home or neighbourhood. These are the points to think about:

• **Disruption.** The disruption starts when you first begin to think about moving – looking for somewhere else to live, and dealing with estate agents, especially if you are buying and selling. Except for the lucky few for whom everything goes smoothly, most people have some ups and downs, and sometimes acute disappointment, before they find their new residence. Packing up to move and then unpacking and rearranging in the new home is a big job, even if you are moving from a one-room flat.

• **Change in routine.** Unless you are moving round the corner, every single routine that you have established is going to change: your journey to work, the shops you use, schools, the doctor, dentist, vet, all will either change completely or require reorganisation. More importantly, your routines in the home will have to be relearnt even when everything is in its place. It takes weeks after the move before it feels like home. Until then, every action requires a little more thought than usual: switching on lights, finding your way in the dark, the idiosyncracies of the kitchen and bathroom, knowing where you are when you wake in the night. It is only when matters such as these become automatic that you feel you have really settled in. These changes, although small in themselves, add up to enough to raise your stress levels significantly.

● **Friends, family and social life.** The further away you move, the more likely you are to disrupt the social fabric of your life. Friendships built on proximity and convenience now have to be maintained with effort, and even more effort has to be put into forming relationships in your new area. This can cause both sadness and worry on top of your feelings of being under pressure. If you have children, they too will feel the move keenly and may be more unhappy than you about what has been left behind. Coping with their emotions is an added strain.

● **Timing your move.** Because of all this disruption, hard work and change, you should time your move carefully if you have any choice in the matter. Pregnant women are advised to wait until well after the birth before contemplating a move. In any case, it is better to choose a calm time if you possibly can, so as to remove the amount of stress you experience.

If you have no choice in when to move, you should plan for the fact that this is going to be a difficult time by making the rest of your life as easy as possible. Don't take on too much too soon and do expect to feel more tired than average. This is good advice even if you are moving at the best possible moment.

! ─────────────── *Task* ───────────────

Home sweet home

There are always mixed feelings when you move even if you are going to somewhere much nicer. This is because you are changing from the known to the unknown, and the place you have lived in holds memories for you and has been the scene of happy or important occasions.

Discuss your mixed feelings about the place you are leaving. It is better to acknowledge them than to ignore them.

!

● **The impact on your relationship.** As we have seen, stressful change can make you nervous, irritable and sometimes ill. You are more likely to have pointless rows at this time over insignificant matters. This soon passes if everything else is fundamentally good between you, but it can show up problems that have been lying beneath the surface of your relationship.

Moving also throws you together as a couple and this can be uncomfortable if you have been used to going along separate tracks. The move itself and decisions within the new home require co-operation and negotiation. It can also mean more time together than usual. You can put this to good use by creating new patterns that will continue to mean more time together.

BECOMING A WORKING MOTHER

Most women take some years off after having children before returning to work. If this is your situation, then the decision to return to work, and the changes this means to you and to your partner and family, constitute a major upheaval in all your lives. The mixed feelings that are involved can contribute to making this a crisis point in your relationship.

As with many of the other crises we talk about in this chapter, what this really means is a change in the balance of your relationship, and compromise and negotiation will be necessary before a new balance can be found. Whenever this happens it is the willingness of both partners to adapt to the changing circumstances that determines whether your relationship gains or suffers. It is during a time of upheaval and change that communication becomes essential, and it can shake you out of any rut that has developed in the way you relate to each other.

We are not going to look at the small minority of women who take maternity leave (a few months off from their jobs) to recover from childbirth before going back to the same jobs. Although going back to work so soon brings its own problems, it is not nearly such a big issue within the relationship as when all of you have come to think of the woman as being based at home and always available to the family.

Why work?

Most women want to return to work because the family needs the money. Finding a job becomes essential if your partner is unemployed or his salary doesn't cover the rising costs of family life. But there are often other reasons behind the decision, and it is the feelings connected with these that sometimes cause the tensions.

- **Money**. Needing extra money for the family is only part of it. Some women find being totally financially dependent on their partners hard. Having to account for everything you spend, particularly if it is on a frivolous extra, can sometimes feel demeaning. Worst of all is having to ask your partner for money when it is to be used to buy a present for him!

- **Children growing up**. Many women think about getting a job when their children seem to need them less, perhaps after the youngest goes to school, or even later when the children have left home. This substantial change in your life causes you to think about other changes you might want to make, and what you want to do with the rest of your life.

- **Status**. Many women, while knowing that looking after their families is a valuable job (and more hard-working and responsible than most paid jobs!) suffer from the fact that 'housewife and mother' is an occupation that carries little status. You might be the busiest person you know in terms of being on call twenty-four hours a day and seven days a week, but when someone asks you what you do you say 'nothing'! A job, any job – even a lowly part-time one – can seem more valued than what you do.

But it is the status of being seen as a person in your own right that it also important. Many women find that years of being identified as so-and-so's wife and so-and-so's mum leaves them little sense of their own independent worth. This is one of the reasons that your confidence can become low. If your confidence is affected, then so is your relationship. Counsellors find that it sometimes helps a woman and her relationship for her to go back to work. They find that you gain confidence from an area of life in which you can be seen and valued as 'yourself' and this confidence improves the balance of your relationship. Any work that takes you out of the home does this – it can be voluntary work as well as paid employment.

The impact on family life

If your family has been used to you doing the bulk of chores around the home and being available to take the children to and from friends, clubs and out-of-school lessons, they might mind or resent all this changing when you go back to work. You will need more help with household responsibilities and chores, such as shopping, cooking, tidying, washing up and so on. Older children are sometimes very good at making you feel bad about this, and you should remember that you are doing them a favour by training them to become used to doing their share, which after all, they will have to do when they leave home.

The impact on your relationship

These practical changes affect your partner too. The younger the children are the more you will expect him to take an equal share in the practicalities of daily life. Some men are more willing than others to do this. However, it often becomes the focus of resentful feelings and you might find yourselves quarrelling about the division of labour. If this is the real cause of friction between you then it is fairly easily sorted out by sitting down and discussing what needs to be done when, and negotiating who does it. This is more helpful than you simply delegating jobs and becoming cross when they are not done. By making time to talk about it the *responsibility*, as well as the work, becomes joint.

Constant rows about housework, or your partner flatly refusing to do his share, are, however, usually signs that the resentments go deeper than this.

Some men are openly against you working, other men may seem pleased about it, but underneath are less happy about the arrangement. It is helpful to understand the feelings that give rise to this ambivalence because it is only when they are openly acknowledged that you have the chance of working through them together.

Underlying all the bad feeling is the fear of change and what it might mean. For you the changes are probably positive and perhaps exciting, and your partner can find this threatening.

● **Fear of change in you.** Your partner has become used to you being a certain way. Going back to work is going to change you in ways that he can't anticipate. Even small or good changes can be alarming when they happen in people you believe you know through and through. As your confidence improves you will relate in a different way to your partner and might expect changes in him too. If your relationship is basically good and already well balanced his fears will soon go and he will welcome changes that make you happy. But if you have been having difficulties or the balance of your relationship has been such that as breadwinner your partner has held the power, an increase in independence or earning ability in you will not be welcomed.

Changes in you, therefore, can make him more aware of the areas in which he lacks confidence.

● **Lack of confidence in himself.** Many women go back to work at just the time that their partners are coming to terms with their own professional limitations. If you have taken a new job that excites you it can bring home to your partner his own dissatisfactions. Men who are unconfident are likely to set much store by being the breadwinners and might feel that their masculinity is threatened by you earning money of your own, even if your work is not particularly high-powered.

It can be even harder if your work is more rewarding, better-paid or of higher status. This was so with Bill, who was a manual worker, and Nadine, who was a secretary. Bill saw Nadine's work as more important because it involved writing and dealing with people – things he wasn't good at. They were having rows because Bill wanted Nadine to give up work. Counselling proceeded slowly because Bill could only perceive the job as the problem. It took some time before he was able to see that his strong reactions stemmed from both his disappointment about not having had a good education and his lack of self-confidence in his own abilities.

• **Fear of the relationship ending.** This shows a lack of confidence in the strength of the relationship to withstand the changes. If your relationship has been difficult or unsatisfying, then your partner might feel that the glimpse of another life will make you want to leave him. Sometimes his partner going back to work triggers off irrational jealousy in a man who had previously had it under control.

This was the situation with Andy and Polly, Polly having gone back to part-time work when her youngest started school. Andy had always been possessive and watchful of Polly when they went to parties, but the thought of her having almost daily contact with other men was more than he could bear. All her colleagues were men, and Andy became consumed with jealousy, convinced that she must be about to have an affair. Polly soon learnt that she could not mention any of her co-workers in a friendly way or tell Andy if she had gone with them to the pub for a lunch-time drink. But Andy went on at her to tell him in detail about her day, trying to catch her out, or make her 'confess'.

It came to a head one day when Polly, after finishing for the day at two o'clock, had to drop some papers in on her boss, who was working at home. He invited her in for a coffee. Andy, who was self-employed, had popped home, expecting to find Polly there. He rang her office to find out where she was, and when he heard that she had gone to her boss's house he went mad. He demanded the address and went round. When Polly realised who was at the door, she begged her boss to say that she wasn't there because she was frightened of what Andy might do. This was duly done, but Andy only pretended to leave. He waited round the corner until he saw Polly emerge. He rushed over and grabbed Polly's boss, and they had a fight in the street. Not surprisingly, Polly lost her job and Andy was more convinced than ever that she had been lying all along. Polly had to drag a reluctant Andy along for counselling. Counselling revealed Andy's insecurities, which were long-standing and made it difficult for him to trust anyone to like or love him – even his wife. He only felt secure in the relationship if Polly stayed at home.

!————————————— *Task* —————————————

Time for yourself

Working mothers are usually so busy worrying about their partners, families and work commitments that they forget to make time for themselves. Doing something for yourself and by yourself benefits everyone, not just you. You will feel happier and more relaxed, which will also help your relationships.

It is good for you to have a regular evening out with friends or at a club or a class that you like. Try to build in some physical activity too: exercise classes, swimming, squash, yoga or dance. Exercise helps counteract the stress in your busy life.

!

Your attitude

The reaction of most women to their partners' or children's displeasure about them returning to work is guilt. If you feel you have no right to put your own needs first at times, or you feel that your partner's and children's feelings are your responsibility, this could be your reaction too.

You might find yourself compensating for these feelings of guilt in the way many other women do – by taking on too much; trying to do everything in the home and for the family as before. This leaves you feeling stressed and overtired. Acting like this might make you feel less guilty, but now *you* are the one who feels resentful and angry. Some women find it hard to let go of the caring role or share it with their partners, however willing the men are. Whatever the reason, doing two jobs – at home and at work – increases stress. This is not good for you or your relationship.

Making it work

There are a number of things you can do to make the transition back to work smoother. There are also better ways of handling your partner's or family's resentment than by becoming a martyr.

● **Timing your return.** It is best to return to work gradually if you have any choice in the matter. This helps rebuild any confidence you might have lost while outside the world of work and allows you to sort out over a period of time the division of responsibilities with your partner and other members of the family.

Going back gradually means you can brush up skills by taking a course, or by doing some voluntary work (which is also helpful experience when you apply for paid work). Outside activities such as these allow your partner to become accustomed to you having commitments of your own.

One counsellor remembers Eve, an unhappy, down-trodden woman who came for counselling because her husband, Rick, was having an affair and she felt too lacking in confidence and self-worth to demand that he stop. During the counselling Eve joined her local National Women's Register group, which gave her an evening out once a fortnight. When someone fell ill, she found herself arranging talks and outings for the group, which took up more time and also meant the occasional weekend commitment. Rick agreed to mind the children on these occasions. Eve had been a teacher before she had children, and the confidence she gained from her group activities spurred her on to take up some supply teaching. By the end of counselling, both the insights she had gained during the sessions and the confidence she had won from her new activities helped her confront her husband. She had been offered a full-time teaching job and she was prepared to take it and leave Rick if matters didn't improve between them. But Eve's gradual re-emergence as a woman with a life of her own and a positive sense of herself had already impressed Rick. The battle Eve had been dreading about her husband's mistress never happened: he just gave her up.

● **Dealing with resentment.** Resentment about housework, harboured by your partner or by your children, should not force you into taking on too much yourself. The best way to deal with this is to recognise that the house is a joint responsibility, not just yours. This is easier said than done, as most women are prepared to take everything on their own shoulders. But doing this is not helpful to any of your relationships, particularly your relationship with your partner. Many counsellors see couples where the woman has become 'mum' to the whole family, her partner included. Although this might work happily for a while – another 'marital fit' – it is not an adult-to-adult relationship, and it can mean limited communication, and behaviour that reduces satisfaction in your relationship. Negotiating joint responsibility for the work around the home, and deciding together who does what – not just you handing out the jobs – is a positive step towards a more equal and balanced relationship.

● **Consultation.** Proper involvement of everyone concerned is one way of dealing with resentment. This means consultation at an early stage: explain your reasons for wanting to return to work and what the implications of this are, good and bad. Even young children should be included and will grasp much of what you say.

!================ *Task* ================

We all live here

The housework, shopping and cooking still need to be done when you go back to work. All the members of the family should be involved in this, for their sake and yours. Even little ones can carry out certain jobs: taking the rubbish out, polishing shoes, putting their own washing in the dirty linen basket, tidying their toys, and so on.

The fairest way to spread the work is to draw up a rota. Many working mothers say that this only works for a while and that all the jobs eventually return to them. This is usually because *they* draw up the rota, and *they* decide who does what when.

A more successful system is to choose an evening when you all draw up the rota together and discuss how it will be administered and who will do what. Start from scratch: ask for suggestions to help you list every job that should be done: not just shopping, for instance, but putting it away, too; not just washing up, but clearing the table. The result will be a very long list, which will show the family how much there is to do. Decide together who will do what on a regular basis, and talk about a system for rotating the worst jobs so no one has to do them all the time.

If the system breaks down, call another meeting to decide what would make it work better.

!

This is not the same as asking permission; you may well have made your decision already, but you are doing your family the courtesy of making them understand how you feel and think. In turn, you must allow them to express their own feelings about this, including the resentments. It is feelings being denied or not 'allowed' that makes resentment fester. Listening to them, and respecting them puts the feelings into proportion.

Talking about it together also helps you see whether there is room for appropriate negotiation. One counsellor says, 'Part of my job is asking: What sort of lives do you want to lead? What are you prepared to work at together? What are you getting from each other? How much do you need to be a person in your own right?'

These are useful questions to discuss with your partner. Once you are in a relationship your decisions need to take into consideration the needs of your partner and any children you might have. This is something that most women do naturally. But it doesn't mean putting your own needs *last*. Each person's needs have equal weight.

• **Co-operation.** With proper consultation comes co-operation. If you think about the issues before they occur, you can work out ways to deal with them before they become problems. For instance, talking about how you will arrange for younger children to be looked after or how you will divide the chores *before* it all happens makes it more possible to find agreed solutions.

If you can do this your relationship will benefit immeasurably. A partner who is actively encouraging and who shares the practical duties is also showing that he understands that your rights and needs are equally important in the relationship.

• **Making time for each other.** With both of you working time together can become even more limited. As we have said elsewhere, it is important to make time for each other, even if it means making a date with each other and putting it in your diaries. Making a date means that you often make more effort with each other during your periods together than before, when you had plenty of time. You might be pleasantly surprised to find that you talk more when you are conscious of the preciousness of time together, and that consequently you feel closer and more satisfied with your relationship.

• **Dealing with his fears.** Jealousy, anger and other difficult emotions are dealt with fully in the chapter on Communication. If your partner seems irrationally set against you working, then most of what is said there will be relevant.

Behind anger and bossiness are likely to lurk the kinds of fears we have already mentioned. Counsellors often find that his jealousy and fear is such that inevitably there have already been problems in the

---

! ─────────────── *Task* ───────────────

We are a couple

With both of you working and with a family to look after, it can be easy to lose sight of the fact that the relationship between you as a couple needs cherishing too. Regard making time together as essential for the emotional health of the family, as well as a pleasure for you. Make a regular date to do things together. Find a baby-sitter and get out of the house for a romantic meal, a good film – or anything else you enjoy doing.

It is also a good idea to arrange for your children to stay elsewhere for the night from time to time, so that you have time alone at home for talking, relaxing and lovemaking without fear of interruption.

!

relationship. The problems can only be sorted out by talking about the feelings behind the current fears and finding from where they stem – usually his feelings of inadequacy and lack of confidence.

It is only when you understand what the real issues are that you can hope to be reassuring. If communication is improved he can talk about what is really worrying him. It is difficult for him to say to you, 'Your job has made me feel threatened and I'm frightened that you're going to go off and leave me behind, or you're going to meet someone else.' To say this he needs to feel trusting, and someone suffering from low self-esteem is much more likely to attack instead.

UNEMPLOYMENT

A period of unemployment, or long-term unemployment, particularly of the main wage-earner, creates great practical problems for you, but it is the emotional impact that we are concerned about here.

The balance of the relationship

When one of you has been the main wage earner, your relationship is balanced in ways that you might not recognise until the job goes. Unconsciously, and perhaps unfairly, more value is put on the partner who is earning most or all of the family money. This is often true when it is the man who brings home the bulk of the money. He is the one who usually has the final say about how the money is to be spent, particularly on extras. He might also be given more consideration in other ways – be expected to do less about the house and allowed to have more time to relax and recover from work. Working outside the home also gives him more freedom of movement.

Losing the job

Finding yourself out of work, for whatever reason, is hard. It is a blow even if it has nothing to do with your abilities and the way you tackled the job. The loss of income is only one factor. Also important is the loss of the main focus of your daily life in the work itself and the structure that it gave. It leaves a large practical, physical and emotional gap. Because of all these elements the result is a swift loss of confidence.

In the first instance your confidence is shaken because you quite simply don't know what to do with your day any more. After a period out of work you are likely to find that your confidence goes for other reasons too. The longer you are out of work the more you fear that you might not be able to find another job, and with that comes the deeper fear that you might not have what it takes to do the work involved.

The impact on your relationship

An emotional crisis such as this is bound to affect your relationship. Its effect can go deep because of the way the balance of the relationship changes in the new situation.

We are now going to look at this in more detail, and particularly at the most common situation: when the man who has been the main wage-earner becomes unemployed. Many of the same factors will apply if it is the woman, or for same-sex partners, but when the woman is the main wage-earner and she loses her job, it is less likely to unbalance the situation at home. Women still, in the main, take chief responsibility for housework and child-care, however busy they are outside the home, and many top-earning women go out of their way to reassure their male partners that this makes no difference to the status of either. It is also a little easier for women to have a spell of unemployment in terms of status, because society still regards this as a normal state of affairs.

Being unemployed

When the job ends you are likely to feel shock, but sometimes also relief if you didn't like the work or the employer. Free time can be welcome for a short period. But once these initial feelings have worn off there are harder issues to face.

● **Loss of status.** A man often defines himself through his work and his earning power. When that goes it is common to feel 'less of a man' even though this is not so. In areas of high unemployment you might feel this less acutely when other men you know are in the same situation. But even when there is no shame attached to being unemployed, there is still the problem of not knowing how to define your role in life.

Similarly, many men feel a loss of status within the family, even when the family is supportive and reassuring. Without the confidence and power that go with working and bringing home the family money, you can feel redundant at home, too. Making more of a contribution towards work in the home can feel like lesser employment and even failure. When your partner naturally expects you to do more to help now that you have more time you might find yourself feeling angry, resentful and under attack.

● **Loss of freedom.** Going out to work and having a life outside the home gives a measure of freedom in itself. Having your own money and the ability to organise your time makes you feel master of your life. Without a job, financial and practical considerations mean you are more likely to be at home without the freedom to do what you want when you want.

● **Dealing with the difficult emotions.** As we have seen, many men find it hardest to express the emotions of weakness and fear. While underneath you might be feeling sad, frightened about your future prospects, and depressed over loss of confidence and power, what you are likely to be showing is anger and resentment at the people close to you. If it is your partner who has been made redundant, you too will be feeling a range of difficult emotions. Alongside sadness and sympathy, you are also likely to feel anger. The situation itself makes you angry. You might also be angry because of the way your partner is reacting. You might be fighting irrational feelings of anger at your partner for being in the situation even if it is not his fault. You, too, might feel fear: fear about the practical consequences and fear about how it is affecting your partner.

Coping together

With difficult emotions being felt on both sides, you have to guard against showing only the angry side and burying the fears and weaknesses.

As ever, talking about the full range of emotions you feel is the best way of dealing with them. It might be hard for the man to express his feelings of fear, loss of confidence and weakness, and the woman might find it difficult to hear him do so. Nevertheless, it is only when these feelings can be talked about that they can be handled.

Both of you might find each other's emotions hard to bear at this difficult time, but burying them increases the tensions between you.

Finding a new balance

If you deal with the new situation by talking together and shouldering the responsibilities together, your relationship has the opportunity to develop a better balance. If the man can safely express his fears and weaknesses and the woman can find new strengths in herself, the relationship can end up in better shape than before, even though it is such a difficult time.

What you both need to realise is that this changed situation requires you both to adapt, and being prepared to do so shows the flexibility that is one of the important constituents of a good relationship.

Using the extra time you have for talking and dealing with the situation together increases mutual respect. You can also do essential work on your relationship, if previously there seemed to be too little time to do so. Malcolm and Susannah came for counselling because Malcolm had become impotent after being made redundant. It emerged in counselling that their sexual relationship had never been very satisfying, and after a period of counselling they entered sex therapy. The impotence turned out to be temporary – the cause was psychological rather than physical – and both of them welcomed the free time they now had during the day to work on sexual tasks and develop their sex life in a new and satisfying way. Malcolm's confidence so increased with the improvement in their relationship that he was able to put new vigour into his search for a job. They also both recognised that they had given each other too little time before, so that counselling opened up communication in other ways. When Malcolm found a job they made a pact not to let the new intimacy disappear, and continued to make time for each other.

Practical issues

The way you deal with the practical problems that arise when one of you is unemployed is a good guide to how well you are coping generally.

Taking decisions together, after proper discussion, shows a real working partnership. These decisions will probably include whether the other partner should look for work, how you should manage money, and how you should share the responsibilities in the home. If the unemployed partner insists on remaining in control of all decision-making, or abdicates all responsibility to the other, your relationship will be unbalanced.

Sharing home responsibilities can be surprisingly difficult. If the woman has been at home as a housewife, she might resent her partner's constant presence, and he might feel like a visitor in his own home. It can be hard for both of you to renegotiate the daily pattern. The woman has to give up her hold on the domestic reins, and the man has to accept that taking his share of the household chores is reasonable in the circumstances. If the woman is out at work, the main burden may now fall to the man.

Few people actively enjoy housework, but a true sharing at this very mundane level is indicative of a well-balanced relationship. When you can swap roles and duties so that both of you can work and both of you can look after the home (although you might be better at some things than others), your relationship is more obviously based on choice than need. If your relationship depends on you taking up very separate roles with clearly defined duties and you find it difficult to step outside these, then problems are likely to crop up along the way.

This will be brought into focus if the man becomes redundant. If both of you believe that his role is to work and his wife's role is to look after him, the home and any children, you will both find the enforced change very difficult to manage. He might sit at home being waited on without any compensating activities. If both of you find adapting too awkward and unnatural, the problems brought on by the redundancy will be increased. On the other hand, if you make changes to the way your relationship operates now, it will stand you in good stead when the unemployed partner finds work once again.

!——————————————— *Task* ———————————————

Rescheduling

If you have been working for many years, it can be hard to decide what to do with your time. There is a natural temptation to do very little, but ultimately this will make you feel worse. Give yourself a 'holiday' if you want, but after this is over, aim to get up early and have a full day.

   Set yourself a timetable: allocate certain days or parts of days to look for work, or for something to keep your hand in – retraining or voluntary work. Make a programme to do any chores that you have been storing up, and make time for hobbies and interests that keep you active. If your partner is not working either, or working part time, also include activities to do together during the week which would normally be impossible.

———

——CHILDREN REACHING ADOLESCENCE——

A household with teenagers in it is a household that has periods of chaos and tension. Adolescents have been compared to toddlers, with their switches of moods, strivings for independence and challenges to your power. This inevitably affects you and your relationship with your partner – indeed all the relationships existing between all members of the household. Losing control of your children as they make the awkward and long transition into adults can churn up all sorts of emotions in you: anger, fear of loss of control, fear of separation, and unresolved conflicts from your own younger days.

   The emerging sexuality of your children can also create a host of worrying feelings in you, which sometimes causes a crisis when it happens. Some parents are disturbed by their recognition that their children are becoming attractive adults and worry that their feelings are incestuous; these worries often stop them showing their children affection and can make them seem stern and rejecting. Others feel so distressed that their children are growing up that they become very heavy-handed, not allowing them to go out with friends of the opposite sex and trying to control their time too severely. Some parents feel jealous of the lifestyle of their children, especially if their own adolescences were less free. This is what is most likely to affect your relationship with your partner.

   Bob and Lee illustrate this well. They had been married for twenty years, and had a son and daughter of sixteen and eighteen, Darren and Emma. They came for counselling because Bob was having an affair.

The problems had begun when the children had started to lead lives of their own. Bob found this particularly difficult, and he and Lee had rowed when she first allowed Darren, at the age of fifteen, to stay out all night at a party. A year later Bob threw up his job and went on a course to learn how to set up his own business.

It emerged that Bob, who was forty-one, had had no real adolescence. At no time had he been free to do as he wanted, to make his mistakes or enjoy his youth. At sixteen, when he left school, he had gone straight into the family firm. He lived at home with his parents, as did all his brothers and sisters, until he married Lee. They had not had sex before they were married, and in retrospect Bob admitted that that was the main reason he wanted to marry Lee – that and leaving home.

When Darren started to stay out at night, and it was clear that he was having sex with his girlfriends, Bob was very disturbed. When Emma brought home her first boyfriend he hit the roof, said that the boy was a punk and he didn't want him in the house again. When Bob gave in his notice at the family firm it was at the same time that Darren was starting to look into what college he was going to try for after school.

Bob met Cassie on the business course. She was twenty-seven, and starting a business of her own. Three months into the affair Lee found out and insisted that Bob should come with her for counselling.

During counselling it quickly became evident that Bob was acting out the adolescence he had missed. Leaving the family firm was almost like leaving home, and Cassie appeared to be a fantasy figure of a girlfriend.

His family had controlled him right up to the present day. When he lived at home they had vetted his girlfriends and had once taken his car away until he gave up a girl they didn't like. They had continued to control him as an employee and he had never been given the position of responsibility that he felt he deserved.

As a consequence any feeling that he had any control over his own life was almost nonexistent. When Bob married Lee, he was so wound-up sexually that they had difficulty consummating the marriage. Afterwards he had felt trapped by the marriage because he couldn't be sure that he would have married Lee if they had been able to have sex before and if he had been more free in his choice.

Leaving his job and starting the business course had been exhilarating – but also very frightening. It was an act of rebellion, and Bob wasn't sure that he had what it took to make it work. Lee had got into the habit of putting him down, as everyone else in the family did, but Cassie took him seriously. They would talk together excitedly about their business ventures. Lee finding out about the affair burst the bubble.

After a few sessions, Lee dropped out of the counselling, but continued to be involved at home. Much of the work after this concentrated on Bob's lost adolescence, and all the fantasies and plans he had had to stifle. He talked about going round the world, climbing mountains and being free to experiment sexually. He could see that these feelings had been stirred up by envy of his own children. For a while he thought he wanted out of his marriage as well as his family firm. But gradually, as he talked through all his wild and not-so-wild plans, Bob came to see that he didn't want to lose Lee, despite their problems.

Both Bob and Lee came to see that they had to relate differently – as two adults. The pattern they had fallen into was Lee as the controlling and irritated mother and Bob as the sulky child, not allowed the same freedom as 'the other children'. Bob began to realise that as an adult he was free to incorporate some of his visions of adventure into his life: he had started already with his plans to run his own business and some of his more realistic plans were perfectly possible. But when he became prepared to give up the role of the hard-done-by child, he could also see that he must act responsibly: to have other affairs would jeopardise his marriage, and some of the other schemes would imperil his new business. Knowing that he had a certain freedom of action took away the driving need he had to change everything.

Luckily Lee was willing to change too. She welcomed the more grown-up Bob and was prepared to meet him halfway: her controlling ways had been forced on her by Bob's apathy and she gave them up gladly. She was able to participate fully in his new excitement about life, and as she did Bob found that he did not miss Cassie. Sex between Bob and Lee, which had not been good, started to improve. Bob had lost desire for Lee as she had become increasingly in control and 'motherly'. Sex was for lovers, not for mother and child – as they began to relate as equals and partners, so Bob was able to find Lee attractive again.

If you find that as your children become adolescents you are getting on less well as a couple, be sure to examine what your feelings really are. Sometimes the friction in the home caused by adolescents behaving rebelliously is all there is to it. But if their behaviour is causing echoes of restlessness or resentment in you, taking it out on your partner or embarking on an affair will only make matters worse.

You need to talk about these feelings with your partner. Both of you will be feeling disturbed to a certain degree, but perhaps for different reasons. Answer the questions in the quiz You treat this house like a hotel! on p.207 to identify which are the main difficulties for you, and then make time away from the atmosphere of the home to talk them through together. Identifying the feelings won't necessarily banish them, but it will make you less likely to act in unhelpful or destructive ways towards each other. You can also discuss strategies to make you both feel better during this time – which, after all, will not go on for ever.

CHILDREN LEAVING HOME

When your children finally leave home you become more truly a couple again than at any time since your relationship began. But you are very different people from when you first met and were alone together and this can be a lengthy period of readjustment as you make what amounts to a new relationship with each other.

This can be more difficult than you expect, especially if the last few years with nearly grown-up children around have been bumpy and you have been looking forward to them leaving.

As full-time parents your attention has been split by all the other demands on you, and children can take up almost all your time. Family life is a noisy business, which apparently involves a lot of 'communication' – so much so that you may long for some peace and quiet. But when the children leave you can find out that there hasn't been much real communication between you as a couple. Much of your talking together will have been about your children and practical matters in the home. Your own relationship might well have been neglected, or have been last on your list of priorities.

What you find out when the children leave can surprise even you. Some couples maintain that they have only stayed together for the sake of the children, but when that excuse goes they find that the bond between them is stronger than they thought. Other couples have felt themselves to be happy enough, but find this changes when the children go. This is more often the case when the woman has been a contented full-time mother and finds that without the children her life seems empty and the relationship with her partner is not satisfying enough to take the place of what has gone.

How you have coped with the earlier changes and problems which you have undoubtedly met during your life together, and whether you have gained in liking, respect and love over the years is all thrown into focus at this time. When the children leave it can bring up issues that have been lying dormant in your marriage for years.

Geraldine and Lionel are a case like this. Geraldine had not had a job throughout the marriage, but had put her considerable energies into bringing up Janey and Jessica. At the time that twenty-year-old Janey left home for good, Jessica won a scholarship to a boarding school for talented young musicians. Suddenly Geraldine found herself without a role.

Geraldine and Lionel's marriage had always functioned acceptably at a working level, but they had little in common and Geraldine had not been happy with the relationship. Early on she had tried to get Lionel to agree to them making changes that would improve the relationship, but had eventually given up. Lionel knew that she was dissatisfied, but the marriage as it was suited him well. He thought that women were always dissatisfied; his mother had been, and it seemed that all his married friends were in the same situation.

So it came as no surprise to Lionel when, as the children left home, Geraldine began to complain more consistently and unhappily about their life together. With the extra time on her hands she had more leisure for looking at herself, her life and her future. A cold examination showed her that there was nothing of value left, and little to look forward to.

Geraldine signed up for a psychology course at the local college, and it increased her confidence enormously. It also made her feel that life did hold possibilities for her: there were things she wanted to do that were within reach. But not with Lionel. She could see no point in continuing with the marriage.

Lionel was unprepared for this turn of events. It never occurred to him that Geraldine would ever leave him, and he wanted to save the marriage. This was why he was willing to accompany Geraldine to Relate. Lionel found the process of counselling extremely difficult. He had little insight into how their relationship functioned and why it wasn't working. He was resistant to examining his own feelings and to looking closely at Geraldine's feelings, and their relationship as a whole. He blamed the psychology course for all their problems.

But his desire to keep the marriage alive meant that Lionel slowly conquered his resistance to this analysis and, indeed, began to find it interesting. He became painfully aware that he had always acted 'the strong man' when inside he was much more insecure than he had dared acknowledge. It was this insecurity that had fuelled his resistance to the counselling – and his resistance in the past to taking note of anything Geraldine said.

With this understanding came liberation. Lionel felt much better about himself now that he didn't have to hide parts of himself away from Geraldine. He became prepared to make changes in the way he communicated and behaved.

Geraldine, however, was not sure that these changes had come in time. Her desire to make the relationship work was undercut by the resentment and hurt that had built up over the years when she had desperately tried to make Lionel understand how she felt. Now that she knew she didn't need him she couldn't be sure that she wanted him. When they left counselling, matters were much improved between them. Geraldine had agreed to try living with Lionel in the new way for a year to see whether it would work.

!————————— *Task* —————————

Patterns

The patterns of your life change when the children leave home. Represent this in a diagram to show what changes it has made.

Divide a sheet of paper in three. In the top third represent your family life as it was before the children left home, in the middle third represent it as it is now.

Use circles to represent yourself, members of the family and friends who are important to you. You can make the circles any size you want. Put the initials of each person in the circles and place them as near or as far away from you as you feel they are. Consider their relation to each other. Put up to five pluses and minuses in each circle to show how supportive each person is to you (someone who is physically far away might be very supportive).

Use the diagrams to focus on the way your life has changed. Do you like the new pattern? Is there anything you would like to change? Use the bottom third to draw the pattern you would like if you want changes. Discuss your diagrams with your partner.   !

To change or not to change

Making changes in the way that you relate at this time is partly a matter of choice. As we have seen, unless it is forced on you, making changes – however positive – is hard. Even people who recognise at some level that their relationship is not as good as they would like it to be, still trundle on in the same way because they can't face the effort that the alternative would mean. Indeed, some unhappy couples who really have stayed together for the sake of the children continue to do so: they still want to be available for the children, as a family with a family home to which they can return.

This is good policy – parents breaking up can devastate even grown-up children. But using the opportunity to improve your relationship is even better. Grown-up children are more likely to view your relationship objectively and worry if one of you is very unhappy.

Changing the way you relate will have its difficult moments, and the more entrenched the habits you have to break the more painful it will be at times. Fear of what these changes may mean can be inhibiting. You might think, 'If we look too closely at our relationship and try to change it, will we break up anyway?' But communicating properly is always rewarding, and you have the chance to make the rest of your life together happier and more pleasant than what has gone before.

! ──────────── *Task* ────────────

What do we really want?

When you have both retired you are free of the last ties and restrictions that have stopped you organising your life the way that you want.

Have a 'brainstorming' session, where you sit down together and write down everything you can possibly think of that you would like to do given half the chance. This should be fun: don't eliminate anything – write 'fly to the moon' if you want to.

Look again at your list when you have finished and mark the ones that are practical and possible. Make a commitment to do as many as you can – write them in your diary if necessary. Then look at the the ones that are too expensive or impractical for other reasons. Could you modify them in such a way that they become possible?   **!**

──────────── RETIREMENT ────────────

One counsellor spoke of the 'new sweetness' that couples can discover in their relationship when they have lived together for a long time and negotiated the problems and changes that the years have brought.

One of the last critical hurdles to get over is the one of retirement: giving up work when most of your life has been dedicated to it. Even if you have been looking forward to giving up work, it can be difficult to adjust initially. It carries some of the same problems we looked at in the Unemployment section, above: look specifically at the sections on 'Losing the job' and 'Loss of status'.

It is easier for people who have always led a full life outside work with hobbies, things that they enjoy doing round the house or in the garden, and perhaps voluntary work. But if out-of-work hours have been used just to rest and recover from the labours of the week it will make adjustment harder. Finding new and satisfying ways to fill up your days makes the difference between a fulfilling and an unhappy life. This is the same for men and women when they retire. The more you can find to interest and occupy you, the better it is for the continuing happiness of your relationship.

But if the woman has not worked and has always regarded the home as hers, there will be other problems – what has always been her territory now seems to be 'invaded'. Both of you have to adapt to the fact that you are together all the time. For this to work well the woman has to give up complete control of the house and the man must be prepared to do his share in it. This also frees the woman to develop new interests of her own. Separate interests can be as rewarding as interests that you develop together as a couple, they give you something new to talk about together and also allow you to continue to have a healthy sense of yourselves as individuals.

Retirement gives you the ideal opportunity to renegotiate your whole pattern of life, as well as your way of relating. A flexible, open attitude to life and each other now is a sign of youthfulness of spirit. It is never too late to improve your relationship, as a number of cases in this book have shown. Too many younger couples use the excuse of 'no time!' when they are shown ways of making their relationship better. If you have postponed making improvements, start now.

?_____Quiz_____

'You treat this house like a hotel!'

Your children growing up and the way they behave can make you feel a range of emotions. Read the following lists, and tick all the feelings that correspond most closely to yours; sometimes you will find them mixed and contradictory. Discuss what you have learnt with your partner.

THEY don't do as you say; YOU feel:
a) anxious about your ability to control; b) a need to be tougher; c) angry at them; d) a desire to punish; e) guilty: it was the way you brought them up; f) a wish to get away from the family; g) angry at your partner for not helping;

THEY question and criticise you; YOU feel:
a) upset; b) they have no right; c) defensive; d) a secret fear they are right; e) a need to prove them wrong; f) inadequate; g) it doesn't bother you

THEY are becoming very attractive; YOU feel:
a) proud; b) unattractive and past it; c) need to prove you are still attractive; d) uncomfortable with them; e) anxious about their safety (with the opposite sex and adult strangers); f) disgusted by the way they look; g) sad about their lost childhood

_____?

6

SEX

Sex within a loving relationship deserves a chapter to itself, although giving it a separate section can make it seem separate from the rest of your relationship, when really the two cannot be divided. Except for certain conditions (which are dealt with later), your sex life acts as a mirror to your life together: if things go wrong in other areas your sex life will usually suffer too. All the chapters so far have included examples of couples whose sex life was affected by other seemingly unrelated matters, and in this one it will be seen that many matters that cause concern in your sex life are connected to issues we have looked at in other chapters.

Many books have been written about sex: its problems, its joys and how to make it better. A few of the best are mentioned in the Further Help section. This chapter can't cover every aspect of sex, or go into details about the treatment of sexual problems that need sensitive, professional help. What it can do is look at your sex life in the context of your relationship and how it changes over the years. It will also look at some of the dissatisfactions and worries that commonly arise – some of which can cause problems severe enough to make you want to part, others can make you feel disappointed or unfulfilled sexually, yet otherwise leave your relationship unaffected.

The tasks and quizzes in this chapter are designed to make you understand your own and your partner's sexuality better. They can also help improve the quality of your sex life and suggest changes that might help you feel better about it. The tasks suggested here, some of them similar to those used in sex therapy, appear simple, but they are the hardest in the book. They require communication between you to be good – sex is, after all, communication in its most intimate form. Even couples who communicate well in other areas can find it difficult to talk to each other about sex and each other's needs, or carry out the physical tasks that improve knowledge of each other's individual preferences.

So, it won't be surprising if you and your partner get held up when you decide to carry out some of the tasks. Approach them in the spirit of fun and experiment: see what happens. As one therapist says to couples, 'Just get through it and then curl up together and chat – even if it's only to say thank goodness that's over!' If they are difficult or disturbing,

!————————*Task*————————

Vocabulary

Together make a list of all the other words that you can think of for the following words: Penis, testicles, vagina, breasts, sexual intercourse, masturbation, orgasm, oral sex, anal sex.

Include any private words that were used in your family or that you have made up between you.

Discuss which words you prefer and why. What are the reasons you don't like some of the other words? Decide between you which words you are going to use to talk about sex together. **!**

stop. You might then want to consider counselling. As the therapist says, sexual difficulties are common: 'I often see young, attractive couples who come in with a sense of shame. They think they are the only people not having a sensational sex life. I ask them who knows that they are having problems, and they say no one does. I say, "Quite! Most people don't talk about it but it's much more common than you think." I see them visibly relax to know that they are not alone.'

————TYPES OF SEXUAL PROBLEMS————

Sexual problems are divided into 'primary' and 'secondary'. There are two interpretations of this: primary can mean that the rest of your relationship is good except for the sex, which is the primary problem. In this context, secondary means that the sex problem is one of a number of other problems as well. Primary sex problems can also mean those that you have always had (impotence, inability to have an orgasm), and secondary can mean those that have arisen later, after you have experienced satisfactory sex.

Broadly speaking men's problems divide into ejaculatory dysfunctions: either 'premature', when you come too soon or 'retarded', when you can't come when you want to; and erectile problems: when you can't get an erection at all or not on certain occasions. Women's problems divide into vaginismus: tenseness of the vagina so that penetration is impossible and orgasmic dysfunctions. The latter are pre-orgasmic – you have never had an orgasm at any time; or random orgasmic – you sometimes do, but not reliably. Both men and women may suffer from dyspareunia – pain on intercourse. These 'technical' problems respond well to sex therapy and are best tackled with the help of a therapist. We will be looking at these briefly at the end of the chapter, where we will sketch out how they are handled.

Both men and women experience problems with levels of sexual desire: not fancying each other, or not wanting sex very often or not at all. These are the commonest problems and the most complex even for a sex therapist to deal with because they do not respond so well to purely behavioural techniques. Tasks can help to find the 'sticking point' – where the problem is – and then the therapist's counselling skills are needed to unravel the psychological elements of the problem. These problems of desire, which most often happen when your relationship settles down and are bound up with your feelings about each other, are the ones we look at most closely in this chapter, specifically lack of desire: 'gone off it', different sexual appetites and the disturbing issue of fancying someone else more than you do your partner.

First we are going to look at the patterns of sex in a relationship, and explore how your own feelings about sex have developed.

A 'NORMAL' SEX LIFE

There is no such thing as a normal sex life. There is a satisfactory sex life or an unsatisfactory one, and you are the only judge of which yours is. Statistics on how often people do it – and when and how – only tell you what is average, not what is normal.

However your sex life relates to the national average, you might consider it too much or too little, boring or exciting – it's how *you* see it that counts. If you and your partner are happy with your sex life then it *is* satisfactory and you don't have to worry about how it matches up to anyone else's. If both of you are unhappy about it, then it is not satisfactory, however 'normal' it appears, and you will benefit by making changes. If one of you is dissatisfied it is a problem for both of you. Your sexual relationship is something you share, and it is unhelpful for one of you to insist, 'I'm all right – it's your problem'. If one of you is unhappy about it and this is ignored it is likely to spread to the rest of your relationship, when it will definitely become a joint problem.

Despite the fact that it is inappropriate to assess a sexual relationship according to how 'normal' it is, beliefs about what is normal continue to float around. In previous decades it was considered 'normal' for a woman to feel no sexual desire and simply submit to the man's. Women who didn't fit this stereotype – who showed sexual drive or pleasure – were looked on with horror as 'no better than they should be'. Similar myths still linger on, passed down within families – that men have strong appetites and that women have to endure sex for the sake of family happiness.

At the same time, however, new theories about what is normal have sprung up since the sexual revolution of the sixties, which can be just as damaging. 'Normal' has come to mean a high sex drive and passionate sexual responsiveness at all times – in both men and women. In some people this raises expectations that high levels of sexual interest should and can continue throughout a relationship, that however long you have been together you should be raring to make love at every opportunity. Alongside this goes the theory that if you don't feel this way it must be because you are doing something wrong: improve your technique, change your personal hygiene or the clothes you wear, lose weight and tone up, and then all will be wonderful. Worse still, it is also believed that if you don't continue to feel a high level of sexual desire then you are with the wrong partner. These myths of normality can put a strain on a relationship that is perfectly satisfactory.

The truth lies somewhere between the two extremes: sex will always be part of a good relationship and should continue to be good and satisfying for both partners – but it can lose its urgency and central place at varying times in a long-term relationship.

HOW SEX CHANGES

When you are with the same partner sex changes over the years, as does every aspect of your relationship. Your sexual feelings for your partner change over time and other issues between you affect the way you feel sexually. Various matters in your daily life also affect the sexual side of life.

Statistics show that British couples on average make love twice a week (remember, average doesn't mean 'normal'). If an 'average' couple were to do this throughout their relationship, in one year they would make love roughly 100 times, in ten years 1,000 times, and so on. Forgetting all the other factors that affect your sex life, you can see that it would be surprising if every occasion were to be as fresh and exciting as the first few.

In other activities carried out with similar frequency and consistency, you aim to become quicker and more efficient over time – to get to the point where you can do them without thinking. Sex is the opposite. To remain a satisfying part of your life it needs time, attention, imagination and care, if not all the time then often enough for it to remain pleasurable and rewarding and not become an unexciting routine (described by one counsellor as the 'Press button A, move to B, twiddle with C' approach!).

Sex at the start

During the early days of love passionate sex is usual. When you are 'in love' your body is much more sensitive in its response to your lover, and in that heightened state we talked about earlier, your senses are more alert too. When you think that everything about your lover is perfect it follows that lovemaking seems wonderful. The sight, sound, smell – even the mere thought – of your partner can be highly erotic. It takes very little touching for you both to feel ready for sex. Sex is frequent and happy. Newlyweds who can't get enough of each other may be amused to read statistics on how often long-married people make love. An average of twice a week can seem laughably little: it will never happen to them.

However, not all people have wonderful memories of their early sexual experiences with their partners, or, indeed of their honeymoon. Lack of knowledge about your own and your partner's body can make early lovemaking awkward and unsatisfying. For some people commitment and stability are essential before they can let go fully and enjoy the experience. Sex becomes better as the relationship settles down.

What inevitably changes, whether your sex life started well or not, is the level of automatic sexual interest in your partner. Most couples start a relationship feeling a high level of desire. It varies from couple to couple, but after some time together you need more specific arousal to feel ready for sex. About this time, sex settles into a less prominent place in your relationship. There comes a moment when one or both of you doesn't feel like making love on occasions and a more relaxed pattern of lovemaking is established. For some people even this is a matter of regret. It would be nice if you were in a constant state of sexual excitement about your partner but you might find it inconvenient – or disruptive – if you continued to feel like this throughout your life together!

What is also common is that the quality of your sex life changes. During courting and in the early days of your sexual relationship all sorts of loving touching is usual. Kissing, hugging, holding hands, stroking hair, cuddling on the sofa – these and other gestures are physical ways of saying that you love and desire each other. They create a tenderness and readiness for sex. Sex in the early days is usually more prolonged, with more emphasis on foreplay and a desire for it to be wonderful for both of you. As we saw in the early chapters, with some couples all this stops abruptly after the wedding or the honeymoon. When these aspects are allowed to disappear, however, it can have a major impact on your sex life and how satisfying you find it.

The other factors that cause your sex life to change

How much you fancy each other is only one element in the changing nature of your sex life. Many outside factors have an impact on lovemaking. All relationships have their ups and downs, and during difficult times one or both of you is likely to feel less loving and less sexual.

Major hormonal changes in women also count, such as during the latter stages of pregnancy, after the birth of a baby, and during the menopause. As we saw in the last chapter, it is very common for women suddenly to lose interest in sex in the months after a baby is born. It takes time for desire to return after the physical upheaval of birth and the tiredness that comes with looking after a demanding baby. Sexual desire is lowered in some women even after they have recovered and have a less stressful routine. Hormones, particularly those released during breast-feeding, dampen sexual feelings.

You aren't always told that this is normal and common, and it can appear to both of you that the woman has gone off sex for ever. This is not so. So long as there are no major problems in your relationship desire returns eventually. If you are patient and continue to show your love for each other – including physically, with cuddles and caresses – your normal sexual feelings return. But at times like this and during other upheavals, lack of good communication between you can have a souring effect upon your lovemaking for a long time – forever, if you don't do something about it.

Stress in everyday life can affect levels of desire in men and women. It is understandable that if you are tense and unhappy about something, be it work, financial problems or family matters, you will find it hard to be relaxed and loving about sex. If this causes friction between you the sexual problem may continue when the other issues have been sorted out satisfactorily.

Even with no major upheavals or problems, life for a couple is busy, and if children come along it becomes more so. For many people sex becomes something to be fitted in at the end of the day – after the news or *Match of the Day,* after the washing up and all the chores are out of the way. Couples meet in bed, tired by the day that has just gone, thinking about everything that has to be done in the day to come. Lovemaking is likely to be weary, rushed and mechanical. Unless you make a decision to remedy this you will feel unsatisfied. You'll begin to believe that sex is all 'a lot of fuss about nothing', or only for those who are newly in love.

ur sex life always change for the worse?

seem from this that the odds against maintaining a satisfactory sex life are stacked against you. Certainly, a happy sex life doesn't just happen – every aspect of a good relationship needs effort and thought. But sex can – and ought to – continue to be a satisfactory and pleasurable aspect of your life together. With the right attitude, and improved communication, it can become better than ever – as we saw in Chapter 4, with Alf and Elsie, whose sex life became good for the first time when they were in their seventies. Relate sex therapists find their work rewarding because when a couple show commitment to improving their sex life the results can be outstanding.

?_____ Quiz _____

Descriptions

These are some of the words that people use to describe their experience of sex. Tick any that are relevant to sex as you have experienced it – in either your current relationship or the past. Then choose five words that describe the kind of sex you would like.

exciting	rude	embarrassing
erotic	warm	cosy
boring	intense	dirty
intimate	loving	mystical
uncomfortable	happy	pressurised
animal	disgusting	fun
depressing	alarming	energetic
satisfying	tiring	painful
exploitative	silly	annoying
relaxing	tense	angry
pointless	thrilling	sensual
unifying	friendly	ecstatic
uncontrollable	slow	memorable
passionate	quick	threatening
frightening	gentle	sordid
compassionate	generous	urgent
primitive	powerful	emotional

You can then go on to talk to each other about the words you have ticked and the experiences they relate to – and to explain why you have chosen your five words.

?

A mature sex life can bring great pleasure, fulfilment and excitement. What it can't have is the particular edge of excitement of the early days: that dizzy lust that was there without either of you having to make any effort. However, when you know someone inside out you have the chance of building a sex life that is much better in quality than it was in those early days, even though you won't be able to recreate the 'can't-keep-your-hands-off-each-other' passion.

Later in this chapter, and in the tasks, you will be told ways to increase the satisfaction in your sex life, no matter how long you have been together. If you rid yourself of the idea that lovemaking is downhill all the way then you will be ready to make the effort to improve your sex life.

The X ingredient that makes a mature sex life better than it was at the beginning is trust. A couple who trust each other are free to explore their own needs and take chances without fear. Trust is as important as early lust in uniting a couple and enhancing the quality of their lovemaking. Trust grows out of good communication – and communication is the key to satisfactory sex, as it is to all that is good in a relationship.

SEX AND COMMUNICATION

There is a pop song with the refrain 'How can we be lovers if we can't be friends?' It is a good question which is relevant to a maturing sexual relationship. Lust can unite for a time a couple who may not even like each other, but this will inevitably fizzle out. An enduring sexual relationship which is satisfactory can only be built if you like each other and feel warm and friendly in each other's company.

Communication is about much more than building and maintaining a friendship, as you will know if you have read the chapter on communication. If you have turned to this chapter first, you should read the earlier chapter too as it is essential to apply the elements in it to your sex life as well.

Briefly, these are the main factors that make good communication essential to a good sexual relationship.

● **Knowing yourselves and each other**. Good communication involves knowing yourself and understanding your feelings – and explaining them to your partner, even when they are difficult and negative. It means allowing your partner to do the same, and making real efforts to understand what makes your partner different from you. Respecting and understanding each other's differences and separateness form the basis for a good relationship.

❛—————Talking Point—————

Turn-ons

Take it in turns to describe to each other what you think the opposite sex finds a turn-on in terms of looks, clothes, manner, sexual touching and sexual acts. The woman should say what she thinks men in general like and the man should say what women in general like.

Don't interrupt – hear each other out until the end and then comment on what you both have said.

❜

This is very important when the matter is sexual. Assuming that you are a heterosexual couple, you have the fundamental difference of being of different genders. Men and women tend to bring different ideas, assumptions and needs to the issue of sex, and you have to share these openly to know how to construct a sex life that takes these factors into account. Even same-sex couples will have many different perceptions about sex, which we look at later in the section on 'Your attitude to sex'.

A sex life that grows without these issues being fully understood is a hit and miss affair. Without good communication you have no framework in which you can bring up matters that concern you when they arise and this can turn them into problems later.

● **Talking about sex**. Many people feel awkward talking about sexual needs, problems and difficulties – or even about sexual pleasure. This is increased if you haven't worked through the difficulty of talking about other emotions and thoughts, as explained in the chapter on Communication.

The difficulty is intensified by certain myths such as that nice women don't talk about sex and what they need, and that men automatically know what women want. These myths are summed up in the basic belief that sex should be good without you having to talk about it.

When sex goes wrong between a couple, both of them often have a good idea what it is they don't like – and how they would feel better about it. But they are barred from telling each other how they feel by embarrassment, and by a misguided belief that it is kinder to keep quiet – as well as by the myth that they shouldn't need to say anything.

If you find talking about your sexual feelings and needs too hard, you are likely to fall into one of the basic patterns of unhelpful communication: making assumptions and believing that your partner should know your innermost thoughts without you explaining them. This means that you don't give yourselves the chance to improve your lovemaking.

● **Uncovering secrets.** When communication between you is poor, many things remain unsaid. When these are important to you they become secrets. Whatever the secrets – undisclosed emotions, events from your past, or things that you have done or are doing that you don't want your partner to know – they form a barrier between you. They signify lack of trust in the strength of your relationship to bear the revelations. Openness and trust are such important ingredients in a relationship that the lack of them can be the main cause of a deteriorating sex life.

This is such a basic issue that Relate therapists are reluctant to take on a couple for sex therapy if one of them is protecting a secret that he or she refuses to share. Before a couple is accepted for sex therapy they are seen separately for 'history taking', during which they talk about their entire life as well as their sexual difficulties. In the course of this one of them might reveal that he or she is having an affair. The therapist encourages this person to tell the partner, or offers to help in the telling at a session when the couple are together. If the secretive partner refuses, the therapist will not break the confidence, but will have to point out that the sex therapy may not be useful. Secrets block the intimacy that is essential to good sex. Other secrets, such as that you were sexually abused as a child or have always faked orgasm, or some other issue central to your sexual feelings, should also be shared if progress is to be made. People usually find it much easier to tell partners their secrets once they have been able to share them with a sympathetic therapist.

● **Dealing with anger.** As we have seen in earlier chapters, anger is usually the direct opposite of an aphrodisiac. Therapists working with couples with sexual problems find that anger – whether it is expressed or unexpressed – is regularly behind the fact that one or both of them doesn't enjoy sex or doesn't want it any more.

On the other hand some people do find anger and aggression erotic – in the early days of a relationship it can add spice to your relationship to have a row and make up by making love. It is especially true of anger driven by jealousy. But this is only the case when the good feelings outweigh the bad. When anger continues to be central in your relationship, bed is likely to be a place that you share without touching, in an uneasy, cold truce – rather than a passionate battleground.

Both women and men are likely to express their anger by going off sex. Some men, however, are able to separate emotions from the act of making love and can want to continue even when they are not getting on with their partners. But most women see this as an insult. If he's not feeling tender enough to kiss and cuddle romantically, she feels used when he still wants sex. Anger can cause sexual misunderstandings because many women need to feel loving and tender before they feel sexy. After a row, a man who is not good at expressing his emotions may use sex as a way of saying sorry and showing love, whereas many women need the row to be made up before they are ready to make love.

Expressing your anger and dealing with the source of it can help resolve problems in your sex life. While the anger remains, as with secrets, it acts as a barrier to a good sex life.

● **Communicating through touch.** Touch is an important part of communication, particularly as a way of conveying loving feelings. Keeping up the habit of making tender physical, but non-sexual, gestures, like cuddling, hugging, kissing, (not just as a prelude to sex) helps to maintain a good relationship between you. Touching like this can carry you through the bad times when sex is the last thing on your mind and also helps to preserve the physical side of your relationship.

Touch and other non-verbal communication are additions to talking and listening, not substitutes for them. Some couples try to express their sexual preferences by shifting their bodies towards or away from a specific touch, or convey their feelings through grunts, moans or sighs. This is fine when it works, but sometimes the message gets scrambled

---

! ================= *Task* =================

Touch

These are ten different ways you can use your mouth and your hands when making love. Can you think of any more? Try these ways on different parts of your partner's body and tell each other what feels good where.

Mouth	*Hands*
Kissing with closed mouth	Stroking
Kissing with open mouth	Rubbing
Sucking gently	Kneading
Sucking vigorously	Pinching
Blowing	Scratching gently
Licking with a soft tongue	Scratching hard
Licking with a rigid tongue	Trailing fingertips
Nibbling	Massaging with knuckles
Biting	Tickling
'Grazing' with teeth	Smacking

!

! —————————————— *Task* ——————————————

How does it feel

Collect together the following things, which feel very different:

Something made of silk, or silky fabric, some velvet, a tea towel, a soft sweater, a piece of kitchen paper, a piece of sandpaper, a magazine, a mug, a towel, an apple, a leaf, a sponge, a powder puff, cotton wool, a piece of soft rubber, a feather, a leather shoe.

Take it in turns for one of you to close your eyes and feel each object as it is handed to you by your partner. Describe to each other what it feels like and whether you enjoy the sensations of touching it or not. Say what it is that you like or don't like about the object.

!

and your partner doesn't know how to interpret your unspoken feelings. This can be frustrating if you don't go on to talk about it. For instance, one therapist tells of a couple for whom sex started to go wrong because the woman hated to make love in the morning before they'd cleaned their teeth. Rather than explain, she would turn her face away from her husband when he tried to kiss her. Later, she became more irritated and would push him away, saying 'Not now!' He felt rejected but didn't know what the reason was.

—————————YOUR ATTITUDE TO SEX—————————

Your sex life with your partner is only partly determined by your relationship. It is also affected by your attitude to sex in general. This varies from person to person because it is built up over the years by a combination of factors: the attitudes to sex in the society in which you grew up; popular culture – the films, books and magazines you see; and, most importantly, how sex was regarded in your family. Often these elements conflict and messages from one are contradicted by messages from another, resulting in confused feelings in you.

● **Sex and society.** What messages you have received from the society in which you grew up depends on where in the world you were born, how old you are, whether you lived in a small town or large city, whether or not the community was religious, and many other factors. There are too many variations within these possibilities to go in to, but it is worth thinking about how your world seemed to judge sexual matters

!——————————————————— *Task* ———————————————————

Him and Her

Write down all the words you can think of to describe a boy or man and a girl or a woman who has had lot of lovers.

Which words are praising words and which are derogatory? Discuss whether you agree with them.

!

when you were growing up, and talking about this with your partner to see how your experiences tally.

Despite many great differences and despite the 'sexual revolution', one view is common to almost all cultures and decades: that is, the sexual difference between men and women. Most boys receive the 'message' that men have urgent sexual needs and that it is right and natural for them to get as much sexual practice as they can. To be a 'bit of lad' is something to be admired or at least accepted. Girls, on the other hand, are admired for being pretty, feminine and good – if they have much sexual experience before marriage one generation will call them 'shop-soiled goods', while another will refer to them as 'slags'. Yet despite the fact that some women feel they are not supposed to gain sexual experience before marriage, they are expected to be ready and responsive immediately after.

● **Popular culture.** The films you see, the books and magazines you read and even the music you listen to, all contain messages about love and sex that colour the way you think about the subject. Many of the commonly believed myths are to be found here, masquerading as truths.

The literature and films favoured by many men draw a picture of the macho man, strong, silent and controlled, a natural sexual athlete. He is immediately turned on by an attractive woman and can make love endlessly and repeatedly, bringing even a reluctant woman to orgasm after orgasm. The women are young and attractive with perfect bodies, but they are interchangeable and ultimately disposable. They are not important in the men's lives.

The men in popular women's literature and films are very similar – forceful, emotionally distant and sexually experienced. They are very attractive, have many women and instinctively know how to pleasure women sexually. The main difference is that when such a man falls in love, the emotional floodgates open. He becomes tender and romantic, uninterested in any woman but the love of his life. The woman saves herself for this great love and the first time they make love she is pitched into incredible sexual ecstasy.

These repeated themes raise expectations in both men and women that can make reality seem disappointing. The pressures on men, particularly, are great, and both men and women can feel that the man is at fault if sex is not wonderful. Both believe that the woman should not have to give her man any guidance as to her sexual preferences – in fact, if she does so, she is aggressive and he is a failure.

This was the case with Ellen, who came for counselling alone because she thought she wanted to divorce her husband. She had been married to George for four years and they had a three-year-old daughter. Matters had been going wrong since they had moved to a new area where she knew no one, and into a grander house that was taking up more of his salary and leaving less for extras. A lot of Ellen's problem was anger at George, for not understanding how unhappy she was and for devoting so much attention to his work. Their sex life had all but packed up.

Counselling helped Ellen see that she had expected George to read her mind: she had never explained to him why she felt so miserable. Although this helped the relationship generally it didn't mend their sex life.

Further counselling revealed that Ellen was more sexually experienced than George, a quiet, shy man who had only had one girlfriend before marriage. Ellen resented the fact that George did not know how to make love to her in the way she liked. It was a revelation to Ellen when the counsellor pointed out that it didn't matter that she was more experienced than George, and that it was good for her to be able to show him what she liked during lovemaking. She was also more socially accomplished, and she began to see that this was also a bonus – it was an area in which he needed her particular talents. These insights made Ellen feel much more confident about herself, so that their relationship – and their sex life – improved radically.

In most aspects of your relationship shared expectations are helpful, but in the area of sex they can be the opposite. If both of you expect sex to be all right without effort – for the man to know what to do

---

Task

The 'X' in sex

When you next see a film together or watch a television programme with sex scenes, talk about it afterwards. Did you find it exciting? If so, what bit of it? Did you find it disgusting? If so why particularly? Did you find it funny or boring or over-the-top? Find reasons to explain how you felt.

automatically and for neither of you to have to talk about your needs and desires – it will be difficult for you to develop a sex life that is satisfactory for both of you.

● **Your family's influence**. Most of your feelings about sex are developed as you are growing up within your family. It starts from the moment you are born and is so much a part of you that it can be hard to disentangle what you feel – rather than what you think – about the subject.

It's not just what your family say about sex that affects the ideas and feelings that you develop. Much more significant are the unspoken messages. How much physical affection you received as a baby and child, how your parents showed affection to each other, how nudity was regarded – these and other aspects of family life are equally important. Whether you were breast-fed, your parents' attitudes to potty-training and how they treated your own early exploration of your body count too. Your parents' attitude to 'doctors and nurses' games, to girls getting their periods and to boys having 'wet dreams' are other factors that affect your thoughts on sex. What your parents told you about sex is relevant when it matches these other messages. If the subject was never mentioned in your house it also adds to ideas about whether it is natural, normal, secret or dirty. Powerful early experiences – such as accidentally seeing your parents making love, or sexual abuse – and how these experiences were handled also help to form your attitude to sex.

One Relate sex therapist tells of the importance of positive messages from your family. She cites the case of a friend who was brought up at a time when 'nice' girls never thought about sex or slept with anyone before marriage. But because of positive family messages in her own life, she felt free to have an interesting sex life before she was married, and went on to have a good and satisfying sexual relationship with her husband, which continues to be an important part of their relationship after thirty-five faithful years.

The 'silent messages' she received while she was growing up were that sex was good. She remembers the loving, affectionate relationship between her parents – her mother hopping on to her father's knee for a cuddle, and their whispers and secret laughter. Although she sometimes felt a bit excluded, she knew that whatever the 'secret' between her parents was, it was something worth having. The single time her mother spoke to her about sex was shortly before her own marriage. Her mother was fifty-seven and she told her daughter that sex had been lovely and an important part of her relationship with her husband – and it still was. She said, 'You shouldn't expect it to be immediately fantastic, but in time you will learn about each other and it will become very good.'

The combination of what she had picked up about her parents' relationship and this one direct statement, which reinforced all she had gathered, gave her the 'permission' to enjoy sex (which many girls lack), as well as the understanding that it needs to be worked at.

In contrast, Diane and Ashley's sex life was marred by the ideas about sex that Diana had gathered while she was growing up. They were in their late twenties and had two children. Ashley wanted a divorce because their sex life was so unsatisfactory. They had had a good sexual relationship before they were married, but Diane now only allowed sex about once a month and although she enjoyed it she was always reluctant. To Ashley sex equalled love, and if Diane rejected his sexual attentions he felt it meant she didn't love him and didn't want his love.

Diane's mother had never enjoyed sex and had made this obvious to Diane. From the time Diane had started seeing boys her father had handed out dire warnings about not getting pregnant and had said that the best form of contraception was saying 'no'. Diane had always been close to her mother, but after she was married her mother withdrew and became cold and distant.

Diane came to understand that she herself connected sex only with having children, so that now their family was complete she felt it was wrong. Sex was also connected with marriage – and it was on her marriage that she seemed to lose her mother's love. Taken together, these views made sex seem a negative and threatening matter and she felt guilty about enjoying it. Once Diane was able to recognise this her attitude began to change. Through counselling Diane was able to see that sex can and should be a pleasurable part of a relationship and that she didn't have to feel guilty. Their sex life quickly improved and Ashley stopped wanting a divorce.

All these different ideas from your family, society and culture combine to give you a unique view of sex, which you might never talk about to anyone, but which ultimately affects the lovemaking between you and your partner. Some of these feelings may be unhelpful and contribute to making sex between you unsatisfying.

If your sexual feelings differ from the messages you received as you were growing up, the result is often guilt. Like Diane, you can feel bad about the fact you enjoy sex if you were brought up to feel you shouldn't, and a man can feel guilty and abnormal if he is not raring to make love to every woman he meets, or whenever his partner wants to. If you are a gay man or a lesbian you may well feel guilty about your difference, as almost all the messages you received while growing up would have reinforced the idea that only heterosexual relationships are normal.

❛ ————————— Talking Point ——————————

The birds and the bees

When did you first learn about sex? Discuss together how and what you heard about sex and what your feelings about it were at the time.

❜

Your attitude to your body

Attitudes to sex are also connected to your feelings about your own body. These feelings usually develop alongside your attitude to sex as you grow up. Good feelings about your body are important in developing a satisfactory sex life. If you feel apologetic about your body – you think it ugly, abnormal or dirty – it is hard for you to be able to enjoy sex.

An example of the importance of your feelings about your body in relation to sex is Angela, who went off sex totally. She hated her husband looking at her or touching her because she felt so negative about herself. Angela wanted sex therapy, but reacted badly to the first gentle tasks to do with exploring each other's bodies in a non-sexual way. On being questioned, she told the therapist that she liked her head, neck, hands and feet, but nothing in between. She saw her body as an ugly, shapeless blob. The sex therapy had to wait while they worked on Angela's feelings about herself.

Anxiety about your body stops you being able to relax sexually or give yourself up to your own pleasure. Women, particularly, are often worried about whether their bodies are 'good enough', and can feel that they are simply too flawed to be attractive. It is common to think that your breasts are too big or too small or too floppy, and to wonder

❛ ————————— Talking Point ——————————

Home and away

How was sex regarded in your family? Talk about the attitudes held by your parents and brothers and sisters and how sex was mentioned, if ever, in the home.

Talk about how sex was regarded by your friends, first at primary school and then when you were a teenager. What was the attitude to sexually active girls? Did it differ from the attitude to sexually active boys?

❜

❛══════════════Talking Point══════════════

Growing up

Discuss how you felt when you started to develop. What did you
feel about your changing body? What did the woman feel when her
periods started? How did the man feel when he started to have wet
dreams? How did your families react to the changes in you?

❜

whether your sex organs are normal or attractive. Men, on the whole,
have fewer worries about the shape of their bodies, but are concerned
about their potency, or the size of their penises. If you worry about your
partner being put off by your body, then you yourself will be put off,
which can affect your level of desire.

If you were sexually abused as a child this can also lead to unhappy
feelings about your body. A common feeling is that you have no rights
over your body, which can make you feel obliged to have sex whether
you want it or not. If the abuse caused you to feel aroused, then arousal
can make you feel guilty and dirty later on in your life. This can have the
paradoxical effect of making you take more sexual partners than you
want in joyless sex, but with the inability to respond to a loving partner
in a good sexual relationship.

If you felt unloved as a child and had less cuddles and affection
than you needed, this can also lead you to feel uncomfortable about your
body.

─────── BUILDING A GOOD SEX LIFE ───────

The ingredients that make up a satisfactory sex life are quite ordinary.
You don't need special looks or talents, only the willingness to put some
time and effort into it. Some of it is work that you do on your own, the
rest is with your partner – all of it should be pleasurable and will
enhance your relationship and your feelings about yourself.

● **Like your body**. As we have seen, liking your body is an important
part of a good sex life. If you have unhappy feelings about your body it
can be hard to change them – but aim for acceptance to begin with. Look
at your body naked – it is not helpful to compare it to others or to look at
it only to find fault. Think of the parts of your body that you do like and
try to feel affection for the parts you are unhappy about ('That's what I'm
like!') just as you feel affection for less than perfect aspects of people you

---
Talking Point
What I like

Take it in turns to describe to each other the aspects you most enjoy in your lovemaking. Include the build-up before lovemaking begins and what happens after it is over.

---

love. See all of your body as being unique and special to you. During sex therapy you will usually be shown some pictures of naked men and women so that you understand what a great and interesting variety of body shapes there are. This can be a revelation if the only nudes you have seen apart from yourself and your partner are carefully posed and lit pictures of 'perfect' young bodies.

● **Learn about sex and how men's and women's bodies work**. Make sure that your knowledge of sex and how bodies work is accurate. A book such as *Treat Yourself To Sex* (see the Further Help section) is good on this as well as other aspects of your sex life. It gives more detailed information than you are likely to have gathered in general reading, or in the average sex-education talk. This information tells you what is natural and normal and how the body changes and reacts during lovemaking, which is helpful when it comes to knowing yourself and understanding the mechanics of sex. Detailed information such as this is always an early part of sex therapy, and many couples discover things that they didn't know before.

● **Learn what gives you pleasure**. The best way to learn about your own sexual pleasures and needs is to explore your body yourself. Both men and women have often been brought up to believe this is wrong, which makes it difficult for them to enjoy sex fully. Knowing the touches and caresses that you like is an important element in lovemaking. Finding out what feels nice when you touch your own body is helpful when you make love with your partner. Knowing what kind of sexual touching you like, and how to bring yourself to orgasm, are also important. This can be hardest for women who have been brought up to believe that it is wrong. If you know what you like you are better able to communicate this to your partner. Sex therapy always includes this element of getting to know your body and how to give yourself pleasure.

● **Be selfish**. This is an important early lesson that sex therapists teach couples, and it usually comes as a great surprise. It means finding pleasure in all aspects of lovemaking, asking your partner for what you want and enjoying the sensations you receive. It also means taking pleasure in what you do to your partner, and in your partner's pleasure during lovemaking. Satisfactory love-making is a healthy mixture of selfishness and generosity: taking what you need and giving your partner what he or she wants. When a woman expects a man to know what to do automatically she is not being 'selfish' in the right way. Selfishness means actively taking your pleasure. This is an important realisation if you believe that a man should 'give' the woman an orgasm. As one therapist says, 'You can give a woman a bunch of flowers or a box of chocolates, but you can't give her an orgasm.' Your orgasm is your own responsibility, something you 'take' by showing your partner how you like to be touched or by touching yourself. Equally, you make the decision yourself whether you want an orgasm – you don't have to have one every time you make love if you don't feel like it.

Ultimately each of you is responsible for your own sexuality and sexual needs. You have to be able to take to enable your partner to give. Some women believe that sex is something they do for their partners, not something that they should enjoy for themselves, while some men only make demands sexually without considering how their partners feel.

● **Learn about your partner's body**. Take time to explore your partner's body in the way you did your own. Find out not just what turns each other on sexually but how every part of your bodies feels when kissed, caressed, rubbed, licked or any other touch you can think of. Ask your partner to tell you what he or she likes and how the different sensations feel. Do the same when it is your turn.

● **Discover what you like best together**. Each person's experience of sex is individual. What turns one person on will not necessarily do the same for another. What turns you on during one sexual encounter will not necessarily work the next time. If you have had a lot of sexual experience you will have some idea about what you like, but experience with others will not tell you all you need to know about your current partner. Building a satisfactory sex life involves experimenting with the many different ways of making love and pleasing each other to find the variations that you both like. It is a combination of all the ingredients that have gone before: knowing what you like and telling your partner. Finding out what your partner likes by listening and experimentation, and not feeling awkward about explaining what you don't like and why.

The best way of doing this is to tell your partner how you feel about lovemaking. If something feels nice, tell your partner and explain why you like the sensation. If there is an aspect that you don't like, again say why. It is unhelpful to say, 'don't do that!', or 'I hate that', but it *is* helpful to explain what it is you don't like – 'When you touch me like that it tickles', or 'I'm very sensitive there and only the lightest touch feels nice,' – and to go on to explain what would make it better, 'If you touched me more firmly/gently (or whatever) I think I would like it'.

● **Give yourselves time**. In the early days most couples make time for lovemaking. You need to continue to do this if your sex life is to remain satisfactory. You need time to ensure arousal for both of you, with plenty of intimate touching and foreplay before sexual intercourse. Time together after making love is equally important, when you lie together enjoying the feelings of tenderness and closeness – an intimate occasion when it is possible to talk about many matters.

In an increasingly busy life this often means making a date for lovemaking, and creating time and space for sex so that it is not just fitted in at the end of a tiring day.

● **Be flexible**. A satisfactory sex life is changeable. Flexibility means recognising that it will be different on different occasions. Sometimes it will be quiet, low-key and over quite quickly, at other times it will be a major happening, memorable for both of you.

Sex therapists like to use the comparison with food: eating and sex are both controlled by appetites and variety is an important element in retaining interest. The same meal day after day would be boring. At some times you are going to be hungrier than at others. Sometimes one of you will be ravenous, and the other will only feel moderately peckish. Sometimes you'll both be in the mood for an elaborate three-course meal, at other times a sandwich on the run will do. On occasions one of you will want to eat and the other will say, 'I'm not hungry, but I'll keep you company'. A banquet will take much more time, attention, planning and care than a ready-prepared dish that you heat through in the microwave.

! ─────────── *Task* ───────────

Let's do it!

Talk about different ways of making love. Is there something you used to do together but haven't for a while? Is there something that you have never tried but you would like to? This can include sexual positions, sexual acts, use of clothing, and venues other than the bedroom. Agree on one that you would both like to do and make a date to try it some time soon.

!

' ═══════════════Talking Point═══════════════

Fantasy

Describe to each other a sexual fantasy you have had, now or in the past. Then construct a fantasy together that appeals to you both, adding elements that would make it more erotic for you.

,

There will be similar fluctuations in your sexual appetites, which also need loving negotiation. Just as you wouldn't say, 'I'm not hungry tonight so no one gets any food,' so you adapt appropriately to each other's sexual needs. The sexual equivalent of a quick snack makes the sexual banquet even more pleasurable when it happens, and a steady diet of the same sexual encounter time after time will be boring and make both of you lose your appetites.

What makes a good lover?

The ingredients of a satisfactory sex life show that the image many people have of a good lover is inappropriate. Being a good lover is not dependent on having a perfect body or lots of sexual experience or on the ability to make love all night or to have multiple orgasms.

To summarise, you are a good lover if you understand your own body well and are willing to explain and ask for what you want. A good lover is willing to learn what his or her partner wants and out of this to construct various ways of pleasing you both. To be a good lover you also need enough time to practise your skills and use your knowledge together.

Are you happy with your sex life now?

You might be reading this chapter out of interest while feeling perfectly content with your sex life. It is worth giving some thought to keeping it satisfactory. Thinking about your sex life now, while you're satisfied with it, is a way of helping it remain good.

If you are still at the early stage of feeling a high level of desire for your lover, when the slightest touch puts you in the mood for love-making, sex is likely to be good between you. You may genuinely feel that your partner is a wonderful lover. Sex can be very successful without you even knowing why.

But when things calm down you may realise that you've got by with a mixture of luck and lust, and that really you are not very close to knowing exactly what it is that turns your lover on – or that your lover has very little idea what it is that you like.

Now is the ideal opportunity to make sure that what feels good stays good, by becoming more conscious of why it works. It adds an extra dimension of fun to your relationship to agree to identify what is so lovely about it. Taking time to retrace your steps and experiment with precisely what each other likes is thoroughly enjoyable. Saying what you enjoy about sex is important, as is pointing out to each other elements that don't excite you, or that you don't like. Some people feel that it is impolite to do this, but if you say it tactfully and lovingly now, your sex-life will continue to improve. 'I *much* prefer it when you . . .' is one way of expressing a preference. Putting up with what you don't like might seem trivial, but it can affect your pleasurable sexual anticipation, which starts to affect your desire for your partner. Things that niggle in a small way now may assume great importance later. When your sex life is going wrong it is a bad moment to say, 'I never liked it when you . . .'

Catch yourself if you find that you are sliding into a routine with sex. Make an effort to vary matters while you are still happy with your sex life.

Pay attention to the way you communicate in and out of bed. If you let problems fester in your daily life it will affect the happiness you feel when making love. Using sex to smooth over unresolved problems – 'kissing and making up' – only works for a limited time. After that, turning a cold shoulder in bed becomes more common. If you deal with the conflicts when they arise, as explained in the chapter on Communication, bed will remain a place where 'making love' is a literal description of what you do.

Are you unhappy with your sex life now?

The rest of the chapter looks at some of the commonest sex problems and ways of dealing with them. If you are unhappy with your sex life you may find some explanations that can help you.

There are certain matters that need clarifying before you can pinpoint what your problem is – sex therapists do this over four preliminary sessions with clients before deciding whether sex therapy or counselling is more appropriate. It can be useful for you to ask yourself some of these questions.

● **Is it a primary or secondary problem?** The therapist will want to know if it is a life-long problem or whether it has started more recently. If you are a man who has never been able to maintain an erection, or a woman who has never had an orgasm or has suffered from vaginismus and been unable to have sexual intercourse, then the problem is a primary one. These problems are most successfully dealt with by sex therapy and can be hard to overcome on your own.

If these or other problems have only arisen lately then your problem is secondary. Sometimes they are connected to other problems in your relationship, which need to be sorted out first. If the sexual problems remain then they need to be worked on with specifically sexual tasks. Again, sex therapy can help when your own efforts fail.

● **How is the rest of your relationship?** Whether your problems are primary or secondary, to be treated successfully your relationship must be stable and 'good enough'. Working on your sexual relationship can be stressful and if there are other difficulties within your relationship they will start to show. A sex therapist who realises that there are other problems will usually suggest relationship counselling before you tackle the sex side. If you can acknowledge that there are other problems, then you will benefit from rereading the chapter on communication and completing the tasks before concentrating on the sexual difficulties.

● **Could there be a physical cause of your problem?** Certain medical conditions can affect your sex life. There might be real physical reasons why a man or woman has pain on intercourse, and some illnesses affect a man's ability to achieve an erection. Certain prescribed drugs have side effects that can stop a man getting an erection, or can reduce desire and arousal in both men and women. Sex therapists take careful note of any medical conditions and prescribed drugs, and sometimes will suggest a physical check-up or that you ask the doctor whether a prescription can be changed to a medication without particular side effects. You should check with your own doctor about possible medical causes before you assume that your problem is purely a sexual one.

The therapist will also ask about how much you drink. Alcohol affects a man's capacity to get an erection. Other drugs – marijuana, heroin and so on – also affect sexual functioning.

A woman's hormones can affect levels of sexual interest and arousal, especially during the menopause. Hormone levels start to fluctuate before you experience some of the more obvious symptoms of the menopause such as missed periods or hot flushes. Some women whose sex lives have been adversely affected by the menopause find that Hormone Replacement Therapy (HRT) restores desire, as do some complementary remedies. As mentioned earlier, during pregnancy and the months after the birth, hormone levels as well as other factors can cause you to lose interest in sex.

The therapist will also want to know if one or other of you is

!————————————— *Task* —————————————

What do you want from your sex life?

If you are unhappy about your sex life analyse specifically what it is that you don't like. What would make it better in practical ways?

Discuss what each of you could do to improve matters, and make a list. What would either of you find difficult about this new behaviour? Discuss ways you could make it easier for yourselves.

Make the changes one at a time, and discuss afterwards how you felt about each one and whether you want to go on to the next. **!**

clinically depressed – not just feeling low. This too needs attention before the sexual problem can be tackled.

Sometimes a physical cause is uncovered that will mean that sex can never be the way it was between you; for instance, a man might have a condition that means he is not likely to get an erection again. Sex therapy is also useful here. It teaches that penetration is not the be-all and end-all of sex, and that it is perfectly possible to have a pleasurable and satisfying sex life without it.

Even if you don't suffer from a medical condition that affects sexual functioning, feeling physically under par can take away your interest in sex. If you are ill, stressed or very tired it is perfectly understandable that you don't feel like sex at the moment. This is part of the normal waxing and waning of sexual interest and provided everything else is all right it should come back again when you are feeling better.

● **How motivated are you?** Feeling dissatisfied about your sex life is one thing – but are you prepared to put the effort into making it better? Bringing satisfaction back into your sex life takes time and will involve both of you changing some of your patterns of behaviour. If you feel the problem should mend itself or that it is only your partner's responsibility, or your partner would rather leave matters as they are, it is unlikely to improve.

● **Have you got the time – and the place?** Whether you are seeking to improve your sex life through sex therapy or on your own, you do need to make the time to carry out the work properly. Sex therapy involves a weekly meeting with your therapist, as well as time at home to practise. Even if you are tackling the problem on your own, for matters to improve you need to find at least three separate hours to be able to devote to each other during the week. This needs to be quality time – not just fitted in at the end of the day – and time when you know you won't be disturbed.

It also means having a place where you can be private and which you can make warm and welcoming. One therapist tells of an engaged couple who were having sexual problems, but the only place they could do their tasks was in the fiancé's car, so therapy was out of the question.

● **What do you want from your sex life?** In therapy the therapist will ask both partners to say what it is they want from the treatment. These aims are then written down so that the couple and the therapist know what they are working towards. It is also a chance for the therapist to help the couple clarify what they want from their sex life – saying you want it to be 'better' is too woolly – and to see whether their expectations are realistic. For instance, if the couple want the woman to come to orgasm with penile thrusting alone (what one therapist calls 'no hands' sex), it is pointed out that statistics show that the majority of women, while getting pleasurable sensations from penile thrusting, need some touching of the clitoris at the same time to reach orgasm.

Working out in what ways you want your sex life to improve is a good exercise to do on your own. It gives you a framework for discussing your needs and how you feel about your sex life now, as well as what would suit you both in the future. Many couples never talk about this. One therapist saw a couple who were having problems, and during their separate interviews asked how frequently they each would like to make love. The woman said the more often the better – every day if possible. She guessed her husband would be happy with once a week or so. During his interview the husband said he would not miss sex if he never had it again, but he guessed that his wife would like it once a week.

If you reveal a discrepancy in your needs you need to negotiate a compromise that would be acceptable to both of you.

DEALING WITH PROBLEMS

If both of you want to improve your sex life there is a lot you can do to increase your satisfaction. There are usually three parts to a sexual problem: matters from the past that make it likely that you will develop a problem; something within your relationship that has caused the problem to arise; and what's happening now that is causing it to continue. The case of Edward and Simone shows all these factors.

Simone's background predisposed her to have sexual difficulties. She grew up in a tempestuous home – her parents fought dramatically and then spent a lot of time in bed saying sorry and making love. Simone was either frightened by her parents rows, or the embarrassed witness to very obvious sexual contact or passionate noises coming from the locked bedroom. There was no affectionate contact otherwise. Sex became connected in Simone's mind with anger and power: when her mother 'switched on' sexually her father gave in to her in other ways. The idea of sex and her own potential power as a woman was frightening to Simone.

When she married Edward sex was all right for a time, but then the problems started. Edward was a doctor, continually on call. Simone was at home with their toddler, never knowing when Edward would appear or how long he would have to spend with them. She felt that she took second place to his job. When he was at home he was often too tired to talk and would fall asleep at odd hours. The only time he seemed to pay her attention was when he wanted sex, which made Simone feel used. She went off sex totally and only 'gave in' once every three or four months.

The problem was maintained by the fact that when Simone did let Edward make love to her in her unaroused state he would ejaculate almost immediately. There was no pleasure or fun in sex for Simone. All it represented was power: in this case her power to refuse him – the only area of their life together over which she had control.

Relationship counselling helped reduce some of the tension between them. With the counsellor's help they worked out practical ways to make daily life together more pleasant. Edward agreed to structure his life in such a way as to be able to give more time to Simone and their child, and Simone responded by making the home more welcoming – in her misery she had stopped cooking or cleaning. As matters improved between them, Simone became better disposed to the idea of sex – and they went on to work with a sex therapist on ways to improve Edward's premature ejaculation and how to give each other pleasure.

As this case shows, dividing sexual problems into types is somewhat artificial – there is rarely an isolated problem, and more usually an interconnected series of difficulties, some of which must be tackled alone, others together. Nevertheless there is no other way to look at the range of problems than singly. We are going to look most closely at those that are connected with levels of desire.

Lack of desire – 'gone off it'

This is the most common problem. In his book *Sex Therapy* Keith Hawton quotes statistics from one sex therapy clinic that showed that out of 257 women with problems, 52 per cent reported 'impaired sexual interest'. Of the 258 men treated, 6 per cent reported impaired sexual interest and 60 per cent reported 'erectile dysfunction'. As desire is necessary for a man to get an erection, many of that 60 per cent will be men who have lost sexual interest in their partners.

There are thousands more people who have stopped desiring their partners but will not think of seeking sex therapy because they assume it is normal and that nothing can be done about it. But going off sex with your partner shouldn't be considered a normal consequence of a long-term relationship which must be tolerated. Nor should it be taken to mean the end of the relationship.

Desire is the most delicate ingredient in a sexual relationship. Part of it is chemistry: a mysterious cocktail of developmental and hormonal factors that makes you fancy one person and not another. This chemistry is automatic and it is either there or not from the beginning of a relationship. The right chemistry gives a powerful kick-start to a sexual relationship, but it is the most fragile element.

It has often been observed that sex starts in the head. This means that desire can also be stirred by imaginings and fantasies even when you are on your own. There is a large element of fantasy in new relationships, which also makes for a high level of desire at the beginning. Illicitness – feeling that sex is not allowed – also feeds this, which is why some couples desire each other strongly before they are married and then find that one or both of them cools off quite quickly afterwards when sex is expected.

Desire is affected by other factors which add durability to the fantasy and chemical triggers if they are present. But if they are absent or other, negative elements are there, then the initial lust will simply evaporate. All the best elements of love – liking, affection, pleasure in each other's company, trust, intimacy, intellectual rapport and any other positive links – feed desire. In contrast anger, misery, mistrust, lack of communication and other relationship problems sap desire, even when the initial level was high.

Difficulties outside the relationship, such as ill health and stress, can also take away desire, although if the relationship is basically good these can be temporary fluctuations.

The last major factor in keeping desire high – or in making it ebb – is the quality of the sexual relationship itself. Knowing how to arouse each other and give each other maximum sexual satisfaction maintains sexual interest, even when the effects of the chemistry have started to wear off, or even when the chemistry wasn't there in the first place. It is simple common sense that if you know that making love with your partner is satisfying and pleasurable then you are going to look forward to it – and carry on fancying your partner. Equally, if sex between you is poor and unsatisfying you will go off it, however much you used to fancy your partner.

Assuming you have already excluded physical reasons (see 'Could there be a physical cause of your problem?' above) broadly speaking desire is affected by three things we mentioned above: what is happening in your relationship generally, outside factors, and the quality of your sexual relationship. If you have gone off sex it is important to identify which of these factors, or combination of factors, is relevant to you, so now we look at them in more detail.

● **Your relationship in general.** A couple who have been together for some years will know from experience that their desire for each other fluctuates according to the way they are feeling. When everything is going well they feel more affectionate and loving, and this is usually matched by higher levels of desire. During a bad patch sexual interest will often fade as unhappy feelings come to the fore. The first time this happens can be very worrying. For some couples it is when the honeymoon period of being very much in love is over and they experience the hangover symptoms of disillusionment as they become tuned in to the less lovable sides of their partners. This can be accompanied by feeling less turned on sexually by their partners. Most well-suited couples go through this stage and find that desire returns – not at the same pitch of excitement as in the early days, but with a reliable regularity.

Sometimes these 'down' periods can cause problems in themselves. When you don't feel like making love so often, or participate without enthusiasm or your partner turns your advances down flat, it can be unnerving or even shocking for both of you. This is the time to think about what you are feeling and talk to your partner about why your sex life is changing. If you don't, both of you will speculate and make assumptions – often wrongly – about what is happening. If one of you simply withdraws, the other can interpret it as a lack of love, or as the partner having an affair. If this causes both of you to withdraw emotionally from each other a barrier is set up which can become established.

However it starts, some couples get to the point where desire has evaporated never to return. If this is your experience you might find it difficult to know why. You might be able to find dozens of little reasons – personal habits or changing physical shape that you find unattractive – but these are not causes. When you desire someone you find their quirks endearing and attractive. Focusing on small details that irritate you usually masks anger or disappointment on a larger scale. If you are turned off by the partner whom you once desired it can be your body alerting you to problems that your mind is ignoring.

Some of these problems are connected to matters in the past and your unconscious ideas about sex. Sometimes a man will go off his wife after the children come along. The wife becomes 'mother', and mothers, he believes, are not sexual beings. Similarly, a woman who was sexually abused as a child by her father might be able to respond sexually until she has children – especially girls. The husband then becomes 'father' – and fathers, she knows, do dirty things to girls. One counsellor talks about a woman with this problem who froze her husband out when their daughter was born, and wouldn't even allow him to remain in the room when she was changing the baby's nappy.

Other problems, although they might have some roots in the past, are specifically connected to the relationship. If there are issues that are causing tension between you your sex life is often the first thing to suffer. Anger, spoken or unspoken, is one of the main causes of lost desire. If you now do not fancy your partner at all, but can look back at a time when your sexual relationship was good and satisfying, there is almost certainly something else the matter. This is why many couples who come for counselling with a sexual problem and are given help with their general relationship often report that sex is now fine again, even without sexual therapy.

Sue and Paul are a good example of this. For the five years before their daughter was born their marriage was very happy. They had spent that time living abroad, changing countries every six months or so, supporting themselves by teaching English. Sex was a good and important part of their relationship. Paul didn't want children, because his own childhood had been very unhappy, but when Sue became broody he gave in because he loved her. She promised that she would only have the one – and when Harriet was due they decided it was time to settle down.

Sue came for counselling when Harriet was thirteen. By this time her relationship with Paul had deteriorated badly. Their sex life was non-existent, and had been for years. Sue had been desperate for more children, but Paul had stood firm. He was a remote father, and Harriet felt unloved by him: her schoolwork was falling off and she had started to play truant. Sue felt that it was only through her that Paul had any connection with Harriet at all. Sue was now resigned to the fact that her sex life was over and that she would have no more children, but she needed help to cope with her bitterness about Paul's failure as a father and what it was doing to Harriet.

Paul did not come with Sue for counselling, but over a period of time the counsellor helped Sue talk to Paul about her feelings – and about his. He was so terrified of being a bad father, as his own father had been, that he hadn't tried to be a father at all. As the weeks passed he gained confidence and he started to build a better relationship with Harriet. Sue, who was a secretary, retrained to become an infant-school teacher, so that she could incorporate her motherly feelings in her work, and she began to feel much better about herself and her marriage. The counsellor encouraged Sue to reintroduce some of the adventurous excitement that she and Paul had enjoyed in the early part of their life together, and they fixed up to go on a mountain climbing holiday.

Sue only saw the counsellor twice more after the holiday. She was radiant when she returned. The changes for the better in the relationship had brought back her desire for her husband. Sex was really good, she reported – you have to be resourceful and imaginative in a tent!

If there are other problems within yourself or your relationship and you have stopped desiring your partner, then improving communication is the way to start tackling it. Although you will sometimes also need to re-examine the way you relate sexually, better communication will give you a good basis from which to do so.

● **Outside factors**. Your relationship can go through a bad patch for no fault of your own. As we saw in the last chapter, all sorts of outside events can have an impact on you: money troubles, redundancy, a death in the family, poor health and others. These events cause stress, and stress affects levels of desire. Again communication is important. Problems outside your relationship can make trouble between you if you don't talk them through. If going off sex means that you also drop other close physical contact you can feel alienated from each other at precisely the moment that you need to feel your partner's support. If one of you rejects the other sexually without talking about how you feel it can set up a chain of behaviour that leaves you feeling more isolated than ever. The one who wants sex can become resentful so that the other responds by withdrawing more. An outside problem then becomes a relationship problem and your sex life suffers further.

Similarly, if a man once fails to get an erection because he is under stress, ill or has had too much to drink he can feel frightened that he is becoming impotent. It can happen to any man from time to time. But if he worries too much, his fear of failure makes it likely that it will happen again. Some men become aggressive and blame their partners for not being attractive enough. Other men withdraw from all physical contact and become cool so as not to put themselves in the situation of having to perform. Some women react by believing it is their fault, or that their men are having affairs. Both react by losing desire for each other. What started as a minor technical hitch can blow up out of all proportion if the couple don't talk about it, and a problem is set up that becomes entrenched.

● **Your sexual relationship**. The nature of your sexual relationship is a very important element in maintaining your desire for each other.

Some couples form a relationship without the initial chemistry that makes for a high level of desire at the beginning. But if they develop a good sexual rapport they can come to desire each other as much as any couple in a long-established relationship.

However, if you put up with unsatisfying sex at the beginning, continuing disappointment in that area is likely to make all desire disappear in time.

Loss of desire can also happen to couples who started their relationship on a high of physical attraction. The lust this generates can make you sexually lazy. While a relationship is intensely erotic and passionate sex feels terrific, you can't do much wrong sexually and very little technique is needed to make the sex satisfying. When you finally emerge from this period, you can realise that things that you always presumed gave your lover pleasure may in fact be boring, or not liked much. Because your partner seemed to be enjoying it you kept on repeating the same formula. You can be with someone who has little idea how to arouse you or who is sexually passive, and because he or she is new and exciting and you are very turned-on it is wonderful. In the early days you may be prepared to ignore this because sex is generally so erotically satisfying that it doesn't matter. When passion is muted it begins to matter a lot.

At this point some people complain they have gone off sex because of their partners' technique: their lovemaking just doesn't turn them on. They might or might not tell their partners this, but if they do the reaction can be bafflement: 'I've always done it like this so why should there be a problem now?' In fact, although nothing has radically changed in their lovemaking, what seemed to work in the past no longer does.

In many cases this is the fault of poor communication. During the heat of first love every caress is a sexual turn-on. Just being together and touching is erotic. The mechanics of the matter are beside the point. But when first lust cools, technique begins to become more important. If your lover remains convinced that stroking your arm drives you wild, for example, he or she will continue to do it, and not look for other specific ways to excite you. If you have never talked to your partner about what turns you on it is easy to see that a time may come when lovemaking leaves you cold. A couple who, during these early days, talk about what they like sexually and experiment with each other to find out what gives them both pleasure, will be building a sex life that remains good once the early passion subsides. But those who don't do this can find that they feel the moment has passed when they could have said what aspects of sex they enjoyed – or didn't.

Charles and Grace are a good example of this. They had a very passionate few months at the beginning of their relationship. It started to tail off after they had been married for a while, and after their son was born it ceased altogether.

Charles was predisposed to have sexual problems. His strict religious upbringing had taught him that sex was a sin. He had been unable to make love to any woman before he met Grace and he was thrilled and delighted that sex with her seemed fine. As the initial passion wore off Grace received little actual pleasure from sex as both of them were too embarrassed to talk about it and assumed that Charles should take charge and know what to do. Grace enjoyed lovemaking for its warm closeness rather than for sexual pleasure. However, after Charles watched Grace give painful birth to Henry he went off sex completely. All his negative feelings came back. Sex was a sin and it made women suffer. He never touched her again, although in all other respects their relationship was very good – they were like brother and sister. They came for counselling fifteen years after their sex life had ceased. Grace had turned forty and had become uneasy at the idea of spending the rest of her life without sex. They had started to argue about it.

Sex therapy was needed to help Charles change his ideas about sex being sinful and the cause of pain. But in this case they also both needed to learn about sexual pleasure – their own and each other's.

If desire has gone out of your relationship because sex itself was never really satisfying, starting all over again sexually can help. Turning the clock back to the beginning and pretending you've just met and know nothing about each other's sexual needs is a good way. Some of the tasks in this chapter can help you find out more about your sensuality and what turns you on. You can also experiment with the more intense sexual techniques that produce orgasm. In a good, continuing sex life it is helpful to realise that sexual intercourse resulting in orgasm is an aspect of sex, but it is not the only one, nor does it have to be the main goal. Other kinds of lovemaking that are sensually pleasurable are equally important.

Desire levels are also affected by a sex life that has become routine – the 'If we're making love it must be Saturday night' syndrome. Knowing that you always make love at the same time, in the same place and in the same way can be reassuring and comfortable, but the lack of surprise can eventually sap your sexual feelings altogether. Just doing things in a new way injects a surprising element of erotic excitement.

This is the time to remember the similarity with food, mentioned earlier. Even if the routine you have developed is prolonged and technically skilled you will tire of it if there is no variation. Sex therapists encourage couples to develop different ways of making love – it doesn't have to be wild and unusual, as described in certain books, but perhaps four or five pleasurable differences, as simple as taking it in turns to take charge of the lovemaking and varying the time and place.

This can also mean changing your attitude to spontaneity – something that some lovers prize highly. Spontaneous sex, with its suggestion of uncontrollable passion is an attractive idea, but it is not without its practical problems. If you have children or even a moderately timetabled life then the opportunities for spontaneous sex become increasingly rare. By all means grab them when they occur, but do also realise that making a date for sex can be exciting in a different way. The planning and anticipation add a new element. You can choose the time and place so that making love together has the chance to be really satisfying.

Unequal libidos – 'different appetites'

As we have seen, the intensity of early passion always fades. This rarely happens at precisely the same moment for both of you. If you still feel passionately sexual but your partner has become cooler you can believe something is seriously wrong when it might only be a slight imbalance in timing. But if this difference is very marked it could reveal the beginning of a sexual incompatibility that will make you both unhappy if you ignore it.

Perhaps the most difficult to remedy cause of a troublesome sex life is a discrepancy in libido – your sexual needs are different. Some people are far less interested in sex than their partners, not because of any problem, but because it's the way they are. There is no law saying how often you should make love to be normal, but it is helpful for domestic harmony if you both have roughly the same needs.

It requires negotiation and generosity on both sides if your needs are different. Too often it is not talked about. The more sexually active partner makes a move and the other rejects it or puts up with it unwillingly. It is generally believed that men have stronger sex drives than women so a woman whose man wants sex more often than she does might accept it as a fact of life. When it is the woman who has the greater sexual appetite the man can feel that his masculinity is threatened. Whereas a woman can 'lie back and think of England' if her partner demands more sex than she wants, a man cannot make himself perform unless his body is ready.

This is one of the times it helps to define together what you want from your sex life. If you have different ideas on how frequently you want to make love you need to negotiate a compromise. As we said earlier when talking about the comparison with food, no well-meaning person would say, 'You can only eat if I'm hungry'.

What does this mean with regard to sex? One suggestion is that if the man wants more sex than the woman they might agree on one night each week to make love. The deal is that he does not make sexual advances at other times, and she agrees to participate fully when they do make love. When it is the woman who needs sex more often the man might agree to pleasure her in ways other than full sexual intercourse, or to stay by her, supportive and affectionate while she pleasures herself. The aim is to develop an acceptance and understanding of the way you both are, to find a compromise that you can live with that is acceptable, 'good enough', if not ideal.

Sexual attraction for someone else

When you can get into bed beside your lover and desire nothing more than to go to sleep or read a book, when a look or the touch of a hand ceases to be an erotic experience, when sex itself becomes cosy, irregular, unimaginative and rarely exciting it can affect your whole attitude to your relationship.

People who believe that love means maintaining the high level of desire of the early days can think that they have fallen out of love. Others who feel that love must be expressed sexually can feel that their partners don't love them any more. Still others feel that their days of passionate sexual interest are behind them now that they have settled down.

Sex can and should remain good between you. If it has gone off, there are ways of bringing back excitement and playfulness into your lovemaking. But you won't feel that same dizzy lust you felt in the early days. That's intimately connected with the fragile sexual chemistry and newness of love, and the fact that your partner is still an unknown quantity. That's why you can occasionally fancy someone much more than you do your partner at the moment – it's nothing to do with love.

This can be dangerous, even for well-matched couples. If sex was important before it can make them dissatisfied with what is basically a good relationship, and lose the will to put energy into keeping it good. This is the time that some couples break up, or one partner might start to look around for someone else – the person he or she erroneously believes to be a 'true' love, for whom sexual passion will always be felt.

It is about this time that you can rediscover that you find other people attractive. This is particularly disturbing if you believe that loving one person should stop you fancying another. It is seriously misleading if you have previously believed that it must also mean the end of loving your partner.

At some time you are likely to find yourself attracted to someone else. When the feelings are strong you will be confused. What does this mean about your love for your partner? Should you do something about the attraction? While you are alive and healthy you will be attracted to other people from time to time – it's normal. It doesn't mean that you don't love your partner, nor does it mean that you have fallen in love with the new person, but, as with any strong feeling it can be difficult for you to analyse what is going on.

Maria was devastated when she found herself powerfully attracted to a man she met at work. She had married Jim when she was thirty-one and they had been together for five years. It was a decision made with heart and head: he was a lovely man and they were very well suited. She had had more tempestuously passionate relationships in the past but she had never met a man she loved as much as Jim – and she also made a good relationship with his son from his first marriage, who came to live with them.

Wayne was a rep for the company for which Maria worked. He was a couple of years younger than she was, and a notorious womaniser. Maria thought Wayne was attractive the first couple of times he popped into the office, but it was at the Christmas party, when he made a pass at her, that she became obsessed by him. He had kissed her and she had pushed him away, but those few seconds of contact had left her literally weak at the knees. She said she felt as if a powerful sexual switch had been thrown and a current was passing directly between her and Wayne. From then on every time she saw him she was left dizzy with desire. Days when he wasn't around seemed flat. She said that the mere sound of his voice outside her office door set up a vibration within her from which she would take hours to recover.

By the time Maria, without telling Jim, went to see a counsellor, she was in a state of confused misery and elation. She thought she was in love. Jim could never make her feel like this. Wayne had indicated that he was ready and willing to have an affair and would let her set the pace. Could she afford to pass up on something so wonderful and powerful – so fated? If you felt like this wasn't it cowardice to ignore it?

The counsellor says that Maria had been expecting her to take charge – like a mother telling her not to be a naughty girl. Instead, she helped Maria look more closely at the cocktail of feelings that created this strong attraction. Wayne reminded her of her first boyfriend, with whom she had been besotted and who had treated her very badly. She felt that a relationship with him would be intensely sexually exciting, but she also knew that he would soon drop her and that they had little in common. She admitted that her life before Jim had been varied and interesting and she had enjoyed many lovers, but she had often been lonely and the prospect of her future had scared her. Her marriage was stable and happy. She had swapped the fear and excitement of an uncertain life for warm security. She compared the temptation of Wayne to her feelings when she was on a diet and denied herself chocolates. 'I say, "I mustn't have one . . . I mustn't have one . . . Oh yes I will!" Then I eat the whole box.' The counsellor took her through her feelings when she gave in to the chocolates: she felt self-disgust, out of control – the anticipation was always better than the actual eating, which gave her little pleasure. Maria herself immediately made the connection with the way she was likely to feel if she started an affair with Wayne.

They looked at the options open to Maria: to have an affair with Wayne and not tell Jim, to have the affair and tell Jim, to leave Jim, or to make a decision to have nothing more to do with Wayne. None of the options was ideal. Any choice Maria made would involve loss. But as Maria talked through the full implications she came to realise that anything that involved jeopardising her relationship with Jim was the greatest evil. She could see that even a secret affair would inhibit their relaxed and open relationship. She loved him, she loved and felt responsible for his son, and she didn't want either of them to be hurt. Neither did she feel she could endure the pain to her that a relationship with Wayne would involve. She finally decided that the only choice she could live with was forgetting about her attraction to Wayne. She was sure now that she wasn't in love with Wayne. She knew that her strong sexual feelings were not going to disappear, but she felt she had got them into proportion. She decided to look for another job if she found keeping to her decision too hard.

The counsellor urged Maria to think about coming back for counselling with Jim at some point. She felt that perhaps Maria was ignoring issues in their basically sound relationship which could develop into problems. Maria said she was not ready to do so yet, but would consider it.

Sometimes the choice is not so clear cut as Maria's was. The person you are attracted to might seem much more 'right' for you than Wayne was for her. There might be issues making you unhappy with your present partner. But if you are in a committed relationship it is important to look at the implications of acting on your attraction to someone else. Even if you plan to keep it secret there is the possibility of discovery or an awkwardness developing in your relationship. If you are having problems an affair will divert your attention from them – and take you further away from solving them. You have to ask yourself if you are prepared to end the relationship with your present partner. In exchange for passion you stand to give up whatever you have built together as a couple. This means, of course, the relationship between you, but other matters are also affected: your home, your children (if you have any), your network of friends, and your lifestyle together. These are not small considerations. Acting on sexual attraction when you are otherwise involved is dangerous. Only you can weigh up whether it's worth the risk.

CHOOSING SEX THERAPY

It is common to have some difficulty or embarrassment about sexual matters. With the best will in the world you might find that although you and your partner have decided to try some of the tasks in this chapter, you just can't do them – or they bring up uncomfortable feelings for you. That's fine – not everything works for everyone, but it might just alert you to the fact that there is something you need to look at in your relationship, and that you could do with some outside help. Therapy at one of Relate's sexual therapy clinics can help you move on. One therapist told of a couple who, having difficulties in consummating their relationship, had tried to work their way through a book on developing a good sexual relationship. Quite early on they found one of the tasks too difficult and feared that they would never improve their sex life. They did, however, respond well to therapy, with an experienced person helping them talk through the difficulties and changing the tasks to suit them. They went on to improve their sex life radically. The therapist's skill lies in tailoring tasks precisely to fit the couple involved, talking through worries and potential problems in advance, helping couples interpret what is happening, offering encouragement, and unravelling why something is proving difficult. The counsellors in these clinics are referred to as therapists to acknowledge that they have additional extensive training in this specific area of work and that they work in a behavioural way.

If you decide that a sexual problem in your relationship could benefit from sex therapy you will take part in a careful screening procedure, in which the therapist checks out whether it is what you really need.

Part of the therapy usually involves a series of tasks to carry out at home. These sound much simpler than they actually are. Although the methods are basic and easy, they often bring up powerful emotions and sometimes unresolved issues from the past. The therapist's expertise lies in helping you understand and talk through what you are feeling and experiencing – and also in adjusting the pace of the therapy. Sometimes you need to go back a stage, stop altogether, or spend a longer time on a particular task until you are truly happy and comfortable with it.

An important element in the success of sex therapy is finding enough time for it at home. You are asked to make sure you will be not be interrupted, and to organise some of the sessions early in the day or the afternoon. The minimum you are usually asked to aim for is three separate hourly sessions a week. One therapist compares making time for these sessions to learning to play the piano: if you have a lesson once a week but don't practise you'll never learn to play a concerto – or even 'Chopsticks'.

Therapists don't set a new task until you have overcome any difficulties and embarrassments with the last. This can take a few sessions. The therapist compares this careful consolidation of each stage to building a wall. Unless the foundations are solid, and each layer is solidly cemented in, the wall is in danger of collapse; if that happens to you in regards to sex, you will feel a failure and less inclined to try again.

Before you begin a task, you are encouraged to talk it through together, usually with the therapist, as well as at home. What will you find hard? What would make you more relaxed? Anticipating the difficulties is helpful, as is talking it through afterwards to see how you both felt, especially if you were surprised or disturbed about the emotions raised.

The tasks

You usually start with a non-sexual task, designed to help you become comfortable with your body and its sensual feelings. It helps you rebuild a sexual relationship by learning about the pleasure in physical contact. This involves simple, affectionate touching, avoiding the more sexual parts of the body, such as breasts and genitals, without trying to arouse each other, and agreeing not to have sexual intercourse even if arousal occurs. You take it in turns to do this, and are encouraged to tell each other what you find pleasurable – and to enjoy the process of touching your partner as much as you enjoy being caressed yourself.

Many people find this far more difficult than they anticipated, particularly if they have had sexual problems for a long time, which is why it is not recommended that you try it without going to see a sex therapist first.

An example of how sensitive the issue of tasks in sex therapy can be is given by a therapist who set Bruce and Jenny this early task of making time to lie naked together in their bedroom and touch and stroke each other in non-sexual ways. Bruce was to prepare the room, make it warm, cosy and inviting, with music playing, in order to set the scene for Jenny (this was in contrast with their usual pattern of him going straight into sexual intercourse without waiting for her to be in the mood). When they reported back to the therapist they said that it had been a disaster and that they had ended up rowing and not speaking for two days afterwards.

What had gone wrong? Bruce had been afraid that he would make a mistake – choose the wrong music or do something that Jenny would criticise. Before he had finished preparing the room, and some minutes before he was due to call her, Jenny came in carrying a candle, which she suggested Bruce lit. Bruce took this to be a criticism of what he was doing, and they started to argue. Later, when they had half made up, Jenny was stroking Bruce's back as part of the task when she remembered how he used to complain that she was useless at massaging his aching neck muscles. She brought this up and they started to row again. It took some sessions of relationship counselling before they were able to start the tasks again – this time successfully.

When you are comfortable with this first task the subsequent ones become increasingly sexual – involving more intimate touching, still without full sex. Only when this is a happy, pleasurable experience does the therapist suggest that you are ready to resume sexual intercourse.

COMMON SEXUAL PROBLEMS

These are some of the common sexual problems and brief explanations of how a sex therapist might help you to deal with them.

Premature ejaculation

This is the most common male problem, and the most responsive to treatment. If a man always ejaculates before penetration or immediately afterwards then this is premature. This is often connected to him not realising that he is going to ejaculate until it happens. If you both feel that he ejaculates too soon for sex to be satisfying for you both, then there are ways of learning greater control.

One of the most usual ways is the 'stop-start' technique, usually introduced at the stage in sex therapy when the couple are moving on to more specific sexual touching. The aim is for the man to learn to recognise the point of no return after which he ejaculates. When it is the man's turn to be pleasured, he lies on his back, concentrating on the sensations he feels. The woman strokes his penis until he becomes highly aroused. With a word or a touch that they have agreed beforehand, he lets her know that he is close to ejaculating. She then stops stroking and lets his erection subside. After a few minutes she starts the stroking again.

Again, it is rarely recommended that a couple try this without the back-up of sessions talking to a therapist, because a failure to carry it out properly or to deal with the disturbing feelings of hope, fear and anxiety that often accompany it can make the problem more entrenched.

The 'squeeze' technique is another method sometimes suggested by therapists, which should only be necessary if control doesn't develop after several sessions of stop-start.

The woman strokes the man's penis. When he indicates that he is highly aroused the woman firmly squeezes the head of the penis for fifteen to twenty seconds. To squeeze, she holds his penis with her thumb on the underside of the head of the penis below the coronal ridge and with her first and second fingers together on the top of the head of the penis. This will stop him ejaculating. Sometimes he will lose his erection too.

It takes time to be able to co-ordinate this technique and until it is done correctly there may be failures. The woman has to practise how hard she can squeeze when the man has an erection but is not highly aroused.

Only when these techniques are working reliably does the therapist suggest the couple try sexual intercourse again. It is not unusual for the premature ejaculation to recur when they do this, and it can take months before the man is satisfied he has full control. That is why continuing to see a sex therapist can help a couple to understand and manage what is happening to them.

Retarded ejaculation

This is when a man takes a very long time to ejaculate, or is unable to ejaculate at all. The sex therapist asks questions to find out precisely where the problem lies: sometimes he has never been able to ejaculate, or he can by himself but not with a partner, or not during sexual intercourse. The therapist will often suggest that he sees a doctor in case there is a physical cause.

During sex therapy the couple are encouraged to discover how best he likes to be stimulated, and may experiment with lotions and powder to increase his sensations. When there is a psychological element to the problem (connected to messages about sex being dirty or wrong, for instance) the therapist helps him talk about these issues during their appointments.

Erectile problems

This is when the man either can't get an erection at all or not on certain occasions. It is now thought that approximately half of erectile failure has an organic cause. A sex therapist is fully informed of the latest developments in treating this, which include intracavernosal injections, and fildenafil, which is an oral compound. The therapist will also take the man's medical history to check whether he is on medication that affects erectile function, or whether his life-style is contributing to the problem. Again, when the therapist is in any doubt it will usually be suggested that the man consults his GP.

When there is no obvious physical cause, the basic sex therapy tasks, and talking through the emotional issues, can be used to good effect.

Pain on intercourse – dyspareunia

If either of you complain of pain on intercourse, it is important to check that there is no physical reason for this. If investigation shows that the reasons are psychological and, in the case of a woman, she is simply not aroused enough so is not lubricating sufficiently, the sex therapy tasks are used, concentrating on the early tasks until she has learned to enjoy sexual contact and become aroused.

If the cause is physical – a too tight foreskin or reaction to the acidity of vaginal lubrication in men, or internal scarring or other problems in a woman – but sexual intercourse is still possible, therapists will suggest alternative positions or methods that can help.

Vaginismus

This is when the woman becomes so tense that intercourse is not possible. She is usually encouraged to become familiar with her own genitals, and is taught exercises to gain control over her vaginal muscles.

Later, she begins to be comfortable inserting the tip of one of her fingers in her vagina, and progresses to the point that she can insert two fingers and move them without discomfort. Gradually she learns to allow her partner to insert his fingers, sometimes with a lubricant, until this too feels comfortable.

When the couple feel ready for sexual intercourse it is often suggested that they try the position with the woman on top, so that she is in control and can take charge of the movement.

Orgasmic problems

With orgasmic problems the woman is either preorgasmic – she has never had an orgasm at any time, or random orgasmic – she sometimes has an orgasm but it is not reliable. In a tiny number of cases a woman can have an orgasm with intercourse but not by masturbation (a problem, perhaps, for a widow).

An orgasm is not essential for a woman's enjoyment of sex. It becomes a problem if you or your partner think it is and if one or both of you feel disappointed or frustrated if the woman is not experiencing orgasm.

This is usually tackled by masturbation training for the woman alone, so that she knows precisely the touches that can bring her to orgasm. Sometimes a woman needs to use a vibrator for a while to get in touch with the sensations of orgasm before she can learn to do it by manual stimulation alone. Either way, this is followed by the usual sex therapy tasks. The majority of women need some clitoral stimulation as well during sexual intercourse to reach orgasm.

Further sexual problems

There are a range of less common sexual problems – such as phobias, transvestism and others. Most problems can be alleviated to some extent by therapy, or counselling can help you learn to live with them and adapt your relationship to accommodate them.

It takes courage to enter sex therapy or counselling, but living with a problem that is blighting your life and your relationship is the harder option.

? ———————————— *Quiz* ————————————

Show me

These are some ways that people show each other love other than sexually. How many do you do and how often? D = daily; O = often; S = sometimes; N = never

Holding hands; cuddling; calling each other pet names; sharing private jokes; winking; kissing hello and goodbye; kissing at other times; stroking each other's hair; putting your arm round each other; giving each other a massage; chatting on the telephone; writing love notes; spending more than half an hour talking together; pursuing a hobby together; giving each other some free time alone.

Are there any that you would like to do more often? Look at the ones that you never do. Have you ever done them? Would you like it if your partner did them?

——————————————————————— **?**

FURTHER HELP

ORGANISATIONS

Age Concern (England), Astral House, 1286 London Road, London SW16 4ER. Tel. 020 8679 8000

Age Concern (Scotland), 133 Rose Street, Edinburgh, EH2 3DT. Tel. 0131 220 3345

Age Concern (Wales), 4th Floor, 1 Cathedral Road, Cardiff, South Glamorgan, CF1 9SD. Tel. 01222 371 566
Age Concern provides practical advice, information and services for the elderly and retired. Practical help can also be provided, such as assistance with household chores, and help for the housebound. Age Concern also offers funeral planning services and insurance service. Free fact sheets and priced publications are available.

The Beaumont Society, BM Box 3084, London WC1N 3XX
Offers support and advice to transvestites and their partners.

The British Association for Counselling, 1 Regent Place, Rugby, CV21 2PJ. Tel 01788 578 328
An organisation that compiles and publishes a national directory of counselling organisations. Booklets detailing the organisations in your area can be obtained free from the BAC, or in your local library.

British Pregnancy Advisory Service, Action line 0345 304 030
BPAS is a charity giving information, advice, counselling, and practical help for both men and women on issues such as pregnancy, contraception, infertility and abortion. If you require counselling, BPAS will put you in touch with a clinic in your area. BPAS have detailed leaflets on each of their services.

Citizens Advice Bureaux (CAB), address in your local telephone directory.
A service offering free, confidential and impartial advice on benefits and other money problems, rights and problems at work, illness and local organsations that can help with specific problems.

Compassionate Friends, 6 Denmark Street, Bristol B51 5DQ. Tel. 01272 292 778
Compassionate Friends is a charity whose primary purpose is to act as a befriending service to parents whose children have died at any age, under any circumstances. Arrangements will be made to link them with parents who have lost children in similar circumstances but who have come to terms with their loss. Most contact is by telephone or correspondence. There are two special groups. 'The Shadow of Suicide' and 'Parents of Murdered Children'. Compassionate Friends produces leaflets for the bereaved, their friends and professionals.

Cruse Bereavement Care, 126 Sheen Road, Richmond, Surrey TW9 1UR. Tel. 020 8940 4818
A non-political, non-religious national organisation offering help and support for the bereaved. Cruse offers counselling by post, telephone, or personally (this can be at home). Practical advice and information are available through specialists, fact sheets, and a referral service. Cruse holds regular social meeetings and operates a contact list whereby members can get in touch with each other. Cruse has a publication list including leaflets, fact sheets and books.

CRY-SIS, London WC1N 3XX. Tel. 020 7404 5011
An organisation for parents of children who cry excessively. They offer counselling and advice via a local trained counsellor. There are also local support groups, a newsletter and other priced publications.

The Family Planning Information Service, 2–12 Pentonville Road, N1 9FP. Helpline 020 7837 4044
An organisation offering information and advice on all aspects of family planning, pregnancy and sexual health. The service has a wide range of free leaflets and booklets.

FOCUS (Forum for Occupational Counselling and Unemployment Services Ltd), Northside House, Mount Pleasant, Barnet, Hertfordshire EN4 9EB. Tel. 020 8441 9300
FOCUS is a national organisation offering counselling and advice on work issues such as career change, redundancy, retirement, and crisis counselling. FOCUS runs 'Employee Assistance Programmes' whereby counselling is given on any problem (marital, for example) which may be affecting work performance. It also runs Job Clubs for the long-term unemployed. In most instances you have to be referred to FOCUS by your employer, who will pay the fees (you can approach your employer to do this). People who come to FOCUS by themselves can be referred to a counsellor and have to pay fees.

Maternity Alliance, 15 Britannia Street, London WC1X 9JP. Tel. 020 7588 8582
An independent national organisation involved in research and campaigning for better rights and services for parents and their babies. The Maternity Alliance gives practical advice on topics such as monetary benefits, maternity services, pregnancy health advice, and conditions and rights at work. The Maternity Alliance also produces advice leaflets.

Men's Centre Tel. 020 7267 8713
A confidential organisation offering psycho-educational programmes for men who are violent to women.

MIND (National Association for Mental Health) Granta House, 15–19 Broadway, Stratford, London E15 4BQ. Tel. 020 8519 2122
A national charity campaigning to improve conditions for the mentally ill and handicapped. MIND offers support to people in mental distress, from everyday stress to clinical problems. General advice is given over the telephone (2–4.40pm, on weekdays) or by post. Priced publications, advice leaflets, and a newsletter are available.

National Childbirth Trust, Oldham Terrace, Acton, London W3 6NH. Tel. 020 8992 8637. Open office hours.
The NCT is a charity concerned with education for pregnancy, birth and parenthood. There are three main services. Antenatal classes are provided for the last three months of pregnancy. These usually consist of eight sessions of two hours each, and cover all aspects of preparation for birth. Fees are charged, but can be flexible for those in financial difficulties. Breast-feeding help is a free service conducted by telephone or in person. They are also supportive and positive towards mothers who bottle-feed. Postnatal support is offered by local self-help groups. The NCT produces priced publications, leaflets, and a quarterly magazine.

National Children's Bureau, 8 Wakely Street, London EC1V 7QE. Tel. 020 7843 6000
An independent national organisation concerned with the care, well-being and rights of young people and children. The NCB offers an extensive research and information service on a range of issues, including, among others: child abuse; disability; adoption and fostering; parenthood; pre-school education; drug misuse.

National Family Mediation, 9 Tavistock Place, London WC1H 9SN. Tel. 020 7383 5993
NFM's purpose is to help, through high quality family mediation, separating and divorcing parents reach their own joint decisions, focused on the well-being of their children. NFM aims to make family mediation

and supporting services available, regardless of ability to pay, to all separating and divorcing couples.

Parentline-OPUS (Organisation for Parents Under Stress), Endway House, Hadleigh, Essex, SS7 2AN. Tel. 01702 554 782
An organisation that helps parents under stress because of their children. Its aim is to prevent child abuse. It offers friendship, support, anonymity and is noncritical. OPUS encourages parents to help each other and gives them space to share worries and let off steam. Local Parentline-OPUS groups are run by trained parents and offer a befriending service and telephone helpline.

Parent Network, Room 2, Winchester House, 11 Cranmer Road, SW9 6EJ. Tel. 020 7735 1214
A national charity that runs the Parent-Link programme, a support and education system for parents. Parent-Link is a semi-structured course consisting initially of twelve weekly two-hour sessions. It teaches parents how to deal effectively with everyday problems such as untidiness, bad behaviour, bedtime problems, adolescents, etc. It also teaches parents how to help their children develop into confident, independent, caring, considerate and co-operative individuals. The initial sessions lead to regular meetings providing support and further development. A fee may be charged depending on circumstances. There are also workshops dealing with a variety of specific common problems. Leaflets and a newsletter are available.

The Samaritans, address and phone number in the local telephone directory. Available 24 hours a day, every day of the year.
A registered charity that offers emotional support to people feeling lonely, desperate or suicidal. The Samaritans are trained volunteers who provide sympathetic, caring, non-judgmental and confidential support. The Samaritans produce a newsletter and leaflets.

SANDS (Stillbirth and Neonatal Death Society), 28 Portland Place, London W1N 4DE. Tel. 020 7436 5881. Helpline 9.30am–5pm.
A national network of self-help groups and befrienders comprised of bereaved parents. SANDS offers emotional support and practical advice to parents and families whose babies die at birth or shortly after. This help is given by local support groups, telephone, by post, and through leaflets and booklets.

Women's Aid Federation England Ltd. PO Box 391, Bristol BS99 7WS. Tel. 0117 944 4411
Welsh Women's Aid, 38–48 Crwys Road, Cardiff CF2 4NN. Tel. 01222 390 874

Scottish Women's Aid 12 Torphichen Street, Edinburgh EH3 8JQ. Tel. 0131 321 0401
Northern Ireland Women's Aid, 143a University Street, Belfast BT7 1HP. National Helpline. Tel. 01232 249 041 (for emergencies; open 10am–4pm and 7pm–10pm weekdays).
The WAFE comprises a network of autonomous local groups who provide temporary refuge for women and their children who have suffered mental or physical domestic violence. The WAFE operates an open-door policy and tries to ensure that no woman is refused refuge. Priced publications are available in various languages.

Parents at Work, 45 Beech Street, London EC2Y 8AD. Tel. 020 7628 3578. Open Monday–Wednesday; 9am–1pm.
A self-help organisation for working parents and their children providing an information service on all topics of interest to working parents, including practicalities such as child care and pregnant and working mothers' employment rights. It also provides informal support for working mothers and fathers through a network of local groups. Parents at Work gives information on the phone as well as priced leaflets, books and packs.

BOOKS

Becoming Orgasmic – A Sexual and Personal Growth Programme for Women by Julia R Heiman and Joseph LoPiccolo (Piatkus)
A general book about sex, which is particularly useful for women who have never experienced an orgasm. It is very American in style, but the information is comprehensive and helpful.

The Experience of Infertility by Naomi Pfeffer and Anne Woollett (Virago)
An excellent book that combines all the practical information on fertility testing and treatment with a sympathetic understanding of the emotional issues at every stage, written by two women who have been through it all themselves. They also quote extensively from the experience of other men and women.

Families and How to Survive Them by Robin Skynner and John Cleese (Vermilion)
An informative and often amusing book, written as a dialogue between the family therapist, Robin Skynner, and John Cleese. It presents expert and detailed information about the psychodynamics of family life and individual development in a readable form.

The Parent's Book – Getting on well with our Children by Ivan Sokolob and Deborah Hutton (Thorsons)

An excellent, practical book on communicating with children of any age, from babies to adolescents. It is a helpful and reassuring book, with plenty of experiences from other parents and practical exercises.

Men and Sex by Bernard Zilbergeld (Fontana)
A reassuring book for men, and an eye-opening book for women, about what sex is really like for men. It is also a practical book for improving your sex life and dealing with specific sexual problems.

To Love, Honour & Betray: why affairs happen and how to survive them by Zelda West-Meads (Hodder & Stoughton)
A comprehensive look at the mechanics of infidelity, and dealing with the aftermath.

Treat Yourself to Sex – A Guide for Good Loving by Paul Brown and Carolyn Faulder (Penguin)
Easy to read, and reassuring. Practical exercises, 'sex pieces', help you to learn more about your own bodies. It also looks in detail at sexual problems.

What's Your Sexual Style? by Sarah Litvinoff (Coronet)
A look at how your sexual and emotional preferences are affected by your personality – and how you can reconcile your different needs with your partner's.

Working Mother – A Practical Handbook by Sarah Litvinoff and Marianne Velmans (Corgi)
A full guide to being a working mother, relevant to women who go straight back to work after maternity leave, as well as to those who return after years at home with the children. It covers practical matters such as child care for the under-fives and school-age children, housework, illness, and information on employment rights, tax and benefits. It also includes sections on guilt, your home and your partner, and experiences of other working mothers.